PUBLIC HEALTH IN THE 21ST CENTURY SERIES

CONTROLLING DISEASE OUTBREAKS: THE CHANGING ROLE OF HOSPITALS

PUBLIC HEALTH IN THE 21ST CENTURY SERIES

Family History of Osteoporosis
Afrooz Afghani (Editor)
2009. ISBN: 978-1-60876-190-6

Cross Infections: Types, Causes and Prevention
Jin Dong and Xun Liang (Editors)
2009. ISBN: 978-1-60741-467-4

Health-Related Quality of Life
Erik C. Hoffmann (Editor)
2009. ISBN: 978-1-60741-723-1

Swine Flu and Pig Borne Diseases
Viroj Wiwanitkit
2009. ISBN: 978-1-60876-291-0

Home Fire Safety: Preventive Measures and Issues
Cornelio Moretti (Editor)
2009. ISBN: 978-1-60741-651-7

Biological Clocks: Effects on Behavior, Health and Outlook
Oktav Salvenmoser and Brigitta Meklau (Editors)
2010. ISBN: 978-1-60741-251-9

Sexual Risk Behaviors
Luigi Passero and Cecilia Sgariglia (Editors)
2010. ISBN: 978-1-60741-227-4

Expedited Partner Therapy in the Management of STDs
H. Hunter Handsfield, Matthew Hogben, Julia A. Schillinger, Matthew R. Golden, Patricia Kissinger and P. Frederick Sparling
2010. ISBN: 978-1-60741-571-8

MRSA (Methicillin Resistant Staphylococcus aureus) Infections and Treatment
Manal M. Baddour
2010. ISBN: 978-1-61668-038-1

MRSA (Methicillin Resistant Staphylococcus aureus) Infections and Treatment
Manal M. Baddour
2010. ISBN: 978-1-61668-450-1 (Online Book)

Infectious Disease Modelling Research Progress
Jean Michel Tchuenche and C. Chiyaka (Editors)
2010. ISBN: 978-1-60741-347-9

Handbook of Disease Outbreaks: Prevention, Detection and Control
Albin Holmgren and Gerhard Borg (Editors)
2010. ISBN: 978-1-60876-224-8

Firefighter Fitness: A Health and Wellness Guide
Ernest L. Schneider
2010. ISBN: 978-1-60741-650-0

The Making of a Good Doctor
B. D. Kirkcaldy, R. J. Shephard and R. G. Siefen
2010. ISBN: 978-1-60876-449-5

Avian Influenza: Etiology, Pathogenesis and Interventions
Salomon Haugan and Walter Bjornson (Editors)
2010. ISBN: 978-1-60741-846-7

Overweightness and Walking
Caleb I. Black (Editor)
2010. ISBN: 978-1-60741-298-4

Overweightness and Walking
Caleb I. Black (Editor)
2010. ISBN: 978-1-61668-516-4 (Online Book)

Smoking Relapse: Causes, Prevention and Recovery
Johan Egger and Mikel Kalb (Editors)
2010. ISBN: 978-1-60876-580-5

Medicare Advantage: The Alternate Medicare Program
Charles V. Baylis (Editors)
2010. ISBN: 978-1-60876-031-2

Diabetes in Women
Eliza I. Swahn (Editor)
2010. ISBN: 978-1-61668-692-5

Diabetes in Women
Eliza I. Swahn (Editor)
2010. ISBN: 978-1-61668-801-1 (Online Book)

Sepsis: Symptoms, Diagnosis and Treatment
Joseph R. Brown (Editor)
2010. ISBN: 978-1-60876-609-3

Sepsis: Symptoms, Diagnosis and Treatment
Joseph R. Brown (Editor)
2010. ISBN: 978-1-61668-448-8 (Online Book)

Strategic Implications for Global Health
Maria Labonté (Editor)
2010. ISBN: 978-1-60741-660-9

Health and Environment: Social Science Perspectives
Helen Kopnina and Hans Keune (Editors)
2010. ISBN: 978-1-60876-216-3

**Breaking Down Barriers to Care:
Treating Tobacco Dependence in Vulnerable Populations**
John E. Snyder and Megan J. Engelen
2010. ISBN: 978-1-60876-976-6

Controlling Disease Outbreaks: The Changing Role of Hospitals
*Raoul E. Nap, Nico E.L. Meessen, Maarten P.H.M. Andriessen
and Tjip S. van der Werf*
2010. ISBN: 978-1-61668-314-6

Controlling Disease Outbreaks: The Changing Role of Hospitals
*Raoul E. Nap, Nico E.L. Meessen, Maarten P.H.M. Andriessen
and Tjip S. van der Werf*
2010. ISBN: 978-1-61668-739-7 (Online Book)

The H1N1 Influenza Pandemic of 2009
Charles R. Bartolotti (Editor)
2010. ISBN: 978-1-61668-357-3

The H1N1 Influenza Pandemic of 2009
Charles R. Bartolotti (Editor)
2010. ISBN: 978-1-61668-392-4 (Online Book)

**Heavy Metals: A Rapid Clinical Guide to Neurotoxicity
and other Common Concerns**
Kenneth R. Spaeth, Antonios J. Tsismenakis and Stefanos N. Kales
2010. ISBN: 978-1-60876-634-5

The Anti-Inflammatory Effects of Exercise
Pedro Tauler and Antoni Aguiló
2010. ISBN: 978-1-60876-886-8

Physical Activity in Rehabilitation and Recovery
Holly Blake (Editor)
2010. ISBN: 978-1-60876-400-6

**Treadmill Exercise and its Effects on Cardiovascular Fitness, Depression
and Muscle Aerobic Function**
Nuno Azóia and Pedra Dobreiro (Editors)
2010. ISBN: 978-1-60876-857-8

COPD Is/Is Not a Systemic Disease?
Claudio F. Donner (Editor)
2010. ISBN: 978-1-60876-051-0

Research Methodologies in Public Health
David A. Yeboah
2010. ISBN: 978-1-60876-810-3

Diarrhea: Causes, Types and Treatments
Hannah M. Wilson (Editor)
2010. ISBN: 978-1-61668-449-5

Diarrhea: Causes, Types and Treatments
Hannah M. Wilson (Editor)
2010. ISBN: 978-1-61668-874-5 (Online Book)

Scientific and Ethical Approaches for Observational Exposure Studies
Alain E. Hughes
2010. ISBN: 978-1-60876-034-3

Strategic Implications for Global Health
Maria Labonté (Editor)
2010. ISBN: 978-1-60741-660-9

Influenza Pandemic - Preparedness and Response To A Health Disaster
Emma S. Brouwer (Editor)
2010. ISBN: 978-1-60692-953-7

PUBLIC HEALTH IN THE 21ST CENTURY SERIES

CONTROLLING DISEASE OUTBREAKS: THE CHANGING ROLE OF HOSPITALS

RAOUL E. NAP, NICO E.L. MEESSEN
MAARTEN P.H.M. ANDRIESSEN
AND
TJIP S. VAN DER WERF

Nova Science Publishers, Inc.
New York

Copyright © 2010 by Nova Science Publishers, Inc.

All rights reserved. No part of this book may be reproduced, stored in a retrieval system or transmitted in any form or by any means: electronic, electrostatic, magnetic, tape, mechanical photocopying, recording or otherwise without the written permission of the Publisher.

For permission to use material from this book please contact us:
Telephone 631-231-7269; Fax 631-231-8175
Web Site: http://www.novapublishers.com

NOTICE TO THE READER

The Publisher has taken reasonable care in the preparation of this book, but makes no expressed or implied warranty of any kind and assumes no responsibility for any errors or omissions. No liability is assumed for incidental or consequential damages in connection with or arising out of information contained in this book. The Publisher shall not be liable for any special, consequential, or exemplary damages resulting, in whole or in part, from the readers' use of, or reliance upon, this material.

Independent verification should be sought for any data, advice or recommendations contained in this book. In addition, no responsibility is assumed by the publisher for any injury and/or damage to persons or property arising from any methods, products, instructions, ideas or otherwise contained in this publication.

This publication is designed to provide accurate and authoritative information with regard to the subject matter covered herein. It is sold with the clear understanding that the Publisher is not engaged in rendering legal or any other professional services. If legal or any other expert assistance is required, the services of a competent person should be sought. FROM A DECLARATION OF PARTICIPANTS JOINTLY ADOPTED BY A COMMITTEE OF THE AMERICAN BAR ASSOCIATION AND A COMMITTEE OF PUBLISHERS.

LIBRARY OF CONGRESS CATALOGING-IN-PUBLICATION DATA

Available upon Request
ISBN: 978-1-61668-314-6

Published by Nova Science Publishers, Inc. ✢ *New York*

Contents

Preface		xi
Chapter 1	**Introduction**	1
Chapter 2	**Preparing the Health Care System**	7
Chapter 3	**Impact of Avian Influenza in the Netherlands**	9
Chapter 4	**Hospital Capacity**	11
Chapter 5	**Intensive Care Unit capacity**	13
Chapter 6	**Workforce**	15
Chapter 7	**General Practitioners**	17
Chapter 8	**Age Distribution**	19
Chapter 9	**Underlying Disease and Co-Morbidity**	21
Chapter 10	**Mitigation of Pandemic Influenza**	23
Chapter 11	**Containment Measures for Pandemic Influenza**	25
Chapter 12	**Healthcare System Readiness**	29
Chapter 13	**Internal Preparation**	31
Chapter 14	**Business Continuity**	33
Chapter 15	**External Preparation**	37
Chapter 16	**Evidence-Based Management**	41

Chapter 17	Evidence from Focused Modelling: A Case Study from the Netherlands	47
Chapter 18	Healthcare System Readiness	49
Chapter 19	Hospital and Intensive Care Unit Capacity	51
Chapter 20	Workforce	55
Chapter 21	General Practitioners	57
Chapter 22	Age Distribution	59
Chapter 23	Underlying Disease and Co-Morbidity	61
Chapter 24	Mitigation and Containment Measures for Pandemic Influenza	63
Chapter 25	Methodological Considerations	65
Chapter 26	Conclusion	67
Acknowledgement		69
References		71
Index		87

PREFACE

Recent outbreaks of a novel avian influenza A virus (H5N1) in Asia, Africa and Europe were a chilling reminder that another human pandemic may occur any time. Such a worldwide outbreak will cause intense human suffering, disruption of social systems, major economic losses, and greatly burden health care services. Several pandemics during the last century, like the 'Spanish flu' (1918), the 'Asian flu' (1957), the 'Hong Kong flu' (1968) and SARS (2003) prompted health care authorities for preparedness planning. In The Netherlands the risk of pandemic influenza was stressed by the outbreak of H7N7 which led to culling 30 million chickens (one third of domestic poultry), and with one human casualty, a veterinary surgeon. The influenza pandemic alertness was elevated to Phase 3 by the World Health Organization in 2005. In the Netherlands these events forced health care authorities and health care services to draft and discuss national and regional preparedness plans. In November 2007, the northern part of the Netherlands was confronted with a sudden and "mysterious" disease outbreak in an (exotic) animal's pet store. As there was uncertainty about the nature of this sudden outbreak – infectious, toxic or otherwise - all patients were admitted for quarantine and overnight observation to the University Medical Centre Groningen (UMCG), acting as the regional centre for outbreak management and trauma care.

In 2008 a woman died in The Netherlands due to Marburg Haemorrhagic Fever which was acquired during a visit to Uganda. She returned to the Netherlands in good health but after the first symptoms she was admitted to the hospital and deteriorated rapidly with liver failure and severe haemorrhage. These recent incidents emphasise the need for more structured planning and preparation for medical emergencies such as emerging infectious disease outbreaks. Structured planning and preparation for disease outbreaks is not yet common ground for most health services, including hospitals and large tertiary referral centres in affluent countries. It demands commitment from health care services ranging from the level of individual health care workers to government level to provide sufficient strategic decision making and financial resources. It also demands a cultural change in thinking for management and recognizing the ethical impact this has on clinicians and nurses who have to make these decisions. Many clinicians now realize that end-of-life decisions are an integral part of health care which is independent of any specific religious background or culture. With appropriate patient management adequate health care can be provided even during infectious disease outbreaks. Evidence-based medicine and modelling in preparing for disease outbreaks has to be followed by evidence-based management of the health care systems which includes using disease outbreaks models and knowledge about surge capacity on regional, national and international level, to ensure business continuity of the health care system.

Business continuity encompasses ethical decisions (use of surge capacity), finances, and preparation (hospital layout). Decision rules have to be adapted to real-time information updates obtained during the course of an outbreak and exchange of information throughout the crisis is pivotal.

AUTHOR AFFILIATIONS

Raoul E. Nap, MD, MSc, Directorate of Medical Affairs, Quality and Safety, University Medical Centre Groningen, The Netherlands

Nico E.L. Meessen, MD, MSc, PhD, Department of Medical Microbiology, Division of Infection Control, University Medical Centre Groningen, The Netherlands

Maarten P.H.M. Andriessen, MD, PhD, Directorate of Medical Affairs, Quality and Safety, University Medical Centre Groningen, The Netherlands

Tjip S. van der Werf, MD, PhD, Departments of Internal Medicine, and Pulmonary Diseases & Tuberculosis, Infectious Diseases Service and Tuberculosis Unit, University Medical Centre Groningen, The Netherlands

Controlling Disease Outbreaks: Changing role of hospitals
Raoul E. Nap, Nico E.L. Meessen, Maarten P.H.M. Andriessen, Tjip S. van der Werf

Chapter 1

INTRODUCTION

Disease outbreaks are inevitable and unpredictable. The context surrounding an outbreak is always unique and outbreaks are marked by uncertainty and confusion, in the general public, in public services and in public health care. Recent outbreaks with a novel avian influenza A virus (H5N1) in Asia, Africa and Europe are a chilling reminder that another human pandemic may occur at any time in the (near) future [1-22]. Such a worldwide outbreak would cause intense human suffering, disruption of social systems, major economic losses and would greatly burden health care services. Understanding disease outbreaks in general and influenza pandemics specifically requires understanding the pandemics of the 20th century in all their historical, epidemiologic, and biologic context [23].

Since the 1700s, there have been ten to thirteen influenza outbreaks or probable pandemics, of which three have occurred since the beginning of the 20th century: the 1918–1919 Spanish flu pandemic [24-35], the 1957–1958 Asian flu pandemic [36,37] , and the 1968–1969 Hong Kong flu pandemic [28,38]. Another disease outbreak was reflected in the Severe Acute Respiratory Syndrome (SARS) outbreak of 2003 [39-50]. Of the three influenza pandemics, the 1918–1919 influenza pandemic was the most severe, because of the high mortality rate among victims aged 15 to 35 years.

Strains of influenza virus are classified into subtypes by their protein coat antigens haemagglutinin (HA) and neuramidase (NA). Of the 16 HA subtypes known, H1, H2 and H3 are known to have circulated among humans in the past century and, hence most people have gained immunity, attenuating the transmission of the virus. There are three pre-requisites for a viral pandemic to occur: (1) the infectious strain is a new virus subtype which has little or no herd immunity in the population; (2) the virus is able to replicate and cause serious illness and (3) the virus has the ability to be transmitted efficiently from human to human. The H5N1 virus has been shown to have a tropism for human alveolar cells but not to upper respiratory ciliated epithelial cells [51]. Influenza viruses attach to host cells by binding their haemagglutinin to host mucosal sialosaccharides (SA). Avian influenza viruses have affinity to SA-α-2,3-Gal – expressed in airways of water fowl - while human influenza viruses show large affinity to SA-α-2,6-Gal terminated saccharides that are expressed in human airways [52]. This tropism may explain why human-to-human transmission has been uncommon in H5N1 but evidence now emerges that two independent mutations (at positions 182 and 192) in the haemagglutinin molecules independently enhance tropism for human host mucosal cells [53]. The genes of the influenza virus can mutate in two main ways: (1) antigenic drift which involves small errors being incorporated into a virus gene sequence when the virus is replicated and (2) antigenic shift involving an exchange of genes between two types of viruses (e.g. between avian and human forms of influenza virus) when both viruses are present in the same animal or human host cell [19]. As a result of these mutations, the influenza virus changes its protein coat (antigens) and allows for new susceptible non-immune populations to be infected. Through mutations in the viral polymerase gene, there have been gradual adaptations to human hosts and perhaps these smaller ('shift') changes may suffice to eventually cause the virus to cross the species border and become both highly pathogenic and human-to-human transmissible [54]. The H5N1 virus satisfies the first two pre-requisites for a pandemic but has not yet developed the ability to be transmitted easily between humans. A rearrangement or reassortment of avian (H5N1, H7N7) and human (H3N2, H1N1) viruses can cause a new virus that is adapted to human hosts, and therefore highly transmissible. By its new antigenic properties, inherited from its avian ancestry, it would leave humans with no immune protection and therefore this new virus is highly pathogenic. To date such shifts have not been observed with the H5N1 virus and perhaps such reassortments would not result in a deadly and dangerous new virus, as its virulence is yet undetermined [3,55].

Extensive exposure to influenza viruses may also transmit avian influenza viruses, as has recently been shown for influenza A/H11N9 virus among waterfowl hunters and wildlife professionals [56]. In H5N1 avian influenza A, the numbers of cases fallen ill have been documented, but serological information in the general population (as an indicator for the spread of the virus) has been extremely limited. Recently Ci-yong et al reported a positive response of 2.3% in general citizens and a 3.03% positive response in a group with occupational exposure to H5N1 [57]. The sero-conversion rate of H9N2 was 3.7% in general citizens and 9.5% in the occupational exposure group, implying that endemic infections for H5N1 and H9N2 do exist in a Chinese population in the Guangdong Province. Katz et al investigated household and social contacts for the presence of antibodies using neutralising antibody titre and ELISA assays in the first cohort of 17 index patients with confirmed influenza A/H5N1 from Hong Kong. Six out of 51 household contacts of infected humans tested positive, five of whom had also known poultry contact [58]. Sero-conversion after exposure to avian H7N7 influenza A was first believed to be uncommon but this might be explained by the insensitive assay that was used [59]. Dutch investigators developed a serological (haemagglutination inhibition) assay with an unusually low cut-off titre (1:10) that was first validated and proved both sensitive (85%) and specific (100%) [60]. Using this new assay in the H7N7 avian influenza outbreak in The Netherlands in 2003, they showed that 49-51% of exposed individuals had a serological response with only 7.8% meeting the case definition and virological confirmation testing for H7N7-associated conjunctivitis, and; 2% of exposed individuals met the criteria for influenza-like illness (ILI) [59,61,62]. In Hong Kong during 1997, the highly pathogenic strain of avian influenza of H5N1 subtype crossed from birds to humans who were in direct contact with diseased birds during an avian influenza outbreak among poultry [7,8]. The cross-infection was confirmed by molecular studies which showed that the genetic makeup of the virus in humans was identical to those that found in poultry. The H5N1 virus caused severe illness and high mortality among humans. Among 22 persons who were infected, six died [7]. The outbreak ended after authorities culled Hong Kong's entire stock of 1.5 million poultry. No new cases were detected until 2003 when the H5N1 avian influenza virus reappeared, first in China, but later also in several other parts of south-east Asia [63]. It has since spread through migratory wild birds to large parts of Asia, Africa, and Europe [5,20,64-66]. Since then, avian influenza among birds has been reported all over the world, and one of the factors responsible for the spread is the trans-oceanic and transcontinental migration of wild birds [5,20,65-67]. To date, most human deaths from avian influenza have occurred in Indonesia, and nearly all of the human cases resulted from close contact with infected birds [68]. There has been a reported cluster of plausible human-to-human transmission of the H5N1 virus within an extended family in the village of Kubu Sembelang in north Sumatra, Indonesia, in May 2006.

The mechanisms of genetic mutation, antigenic drift, antigenic shift and sero-conversion may produce a new virus that can be easily transmitted between humans and initiate a pandemic. The 1918 influenza pandemic virus was a result of antigenic drift while the 1957–1958 and 1968–1969 influenza pandemic virus was a result of antigenic shifts [32,69-71].

The SARS virus outbreak in Asia saw another type of virus, called the corona virus, which spread widely in a short time. The SARS outbreak is considered to be "minor" when compared to the 1918–1919 influenza outbreak because less fewer than 800 persons died from SARS worldwide whereas 40 to 50 million people died worldwide in the 1918 influenza pandemic. The rapid spread of SARS to Asia, Australia, Europe and North America during the first six months of 2003 illustrates how fast a disease outbreak pandemic can spread across the world. The major reason why SARS was quickly contained was that people with SARS were not contagious before the onset of case-defining symptoms, which allowed effective control measures based on case- identification [39]. A person infected with influenza, however, is contagious before the onset of case-defining symptoms, which limits the effectiveness of isolation of cases as a control strategy for this illness [34].

Avian influenza A (H5N1) viruses cause severe disease in humans, characterized by rapidly progressive pneumonia, multiple organ dysfunction, and high mortality. Poor clinical outcome is associated with high viral load in throat specimens and frequent detection of virus in faeces and blood. The latter finding indicates the potential of the virus to disseminate in humans, similar to what occurs in mammals and birds, which is supported by evidence in autopsy studies of virus in extra-pulmonary tissues such as liver and brain. Deaths from influenza are usually due to secondary bacterial infection, but many deaths during the 1918–1919 pandemic were caused directly by the virus itself. It appears that the immune system in young persons paradoxically went into over-drive while battling the influenza virus, and progressed into an immunologic storm that killed the victims [29]. This was in contrast to the pandemics of 1957–1958 and 1968–1969 which were much milder. There were several explanations for this: The influenza strains were less virulent, the patterns of mortality were more typical for a usual seasonal influenza outbreak (i.e. it was concentrated among the very young and very old) and doctors were able to use antibiotics to treat secondary bacterial infections [72-75]. Experts generally agree that the attack rates (AR; the percentage of the population that becomes ill) of the past three influenza outbreaks in the last century did not differ markedly, and is estimated to be 25% to 30%. Using similar evidence, experts estimate the case fatality rate (the percentage of infected people who die from the infection) during the 1918 outbreak to be about 2.5% whereas the case fatality rates during the 1957–1958 and 1968–1969 episodes were below 0.2% [26].

A number of factors influence the seriousness of a pandemic compared to half a century ago. Factors that suggest that an avian influenza pandemic would be less severe than past pandemics include advances in medicine (i.e. the availability of antiviral medications and vaccines, and international surveillance systems). Factors that suggest than an avian influenza pandemic could be worse than past pandemics include: a more densely populated world;, a larger immune compromised population of elderly and an increased population of chronically sick patients (i.e. AIDS, cancer, transplant patients;), faster air travel and interconnections for people and products between countries and continents which will can accelerate the spread of disease (including trade in poultry and wild birds);[13], increasing global population in which mega-cities in non-affluent countries are without proper hygiene facilities; continuing global destruction of ecological systems and increased scale of food production with increased risk of zoönoses. Also, affluent countries with highly developed and complicated infrastructure are increasingly vulnerable for disruption [76]. The population at high risk for complications due to influenza is expanded because of increased population with chronic illness. During yearly influenza epidemics, groups at increased risk of complications are persons older than 65 years, nursing home residents, adults and children with chronic pulmonary and cardiovascular disorders, and adults and children with diabetes, renal dysfunction, hemoglobinopathies, or immunosuppression [77]. In 2000, approximately 73 million people in the United States were at increased risk of complications from influenza. In The Netherlands this number was 1.4 million people [78].

The threat of an avian influenza pandemic has forced health care authorities and health care services in The Netherlands to draft and discuss national and regional preparedness plans for a pandemic with new human transmissible (influenza) viruses [79-82]. In The Netherlands, one third of domestic poultry –30 million chickens - were culled following an outbreak of H7N7 avian influenza in 2003, with one human casualty - a veterinary surgeon who died from acute lung injury following infection with the virus [61,62]. In 2005 pandemic alertness was elevated to Phase 3 by the World Health Organization (WHO). As of March 11, 2009, 411 cases of human disease have been reported, and 256 of these patients have died [21].

Two recent cases illustrate the involvement of health care authorities, both nationally and locally in disease outbreaks as a result of the preparedness plans developed for avian influenza. On November 5th 2007, the three Northern provinces in the Netherlands were confronted with a sudden and "mysterious" disease outbreak in a animal pet store where exotic animals were kept, leaving 27 people triaged for hospitalization and around 80 health care workers (HCWs) quarantined at the disaster site. Although the last reports from the National Institute for Public Health and the Environment (RIVM) regarded some form of intoxication as the main source of the problem, at the time of the incident there was uncertainty about the nature – infectious, toxic or otherwise – of this sudden outbreak of disease. All patients where admitted to the University Medical Centre Groningen (UMCG), which acting as the regional centre for outbreak management and trauma care. All individuals were detained in quarantine for observation overnight. The UMCG was able to free 30 hospital beds in 4 hours, providing sufficient surge capacity for these patients. To achieve this, patients were transferred from the ward of the department of otorhinolaryngology (mobile non-acute medical and surgical patients) to other wards in the hospital.

In July 2008, Marburg Haemorrhagic Fever was imported into the Netherlands when a 40- year old woman, who travelled in Uganda, returned to the Netherlands. The woman travelled in Uganda from 5-28 June, 2008, and entered caves on two occasions. The first cave was visited on 16 June at Fort Portal. No bats were seen in this cave. She was reportedly exposed to fruit bats during a visit to the "python cave" in the Maramagambo Forest between Queen Elisabeth Park and Kabale on 19 June. This cave is thought to harbour bat species that have been found to carry filoviruses in other locations in sub-Saharan Africa. Filoviruses cause two types of viral haemorrhagic fever: Marburg and Ebola. A large bat population was seen in the cave and the woman is reported to have had direct contact with one bat. The woman returned to the Netherlands on 28 June in good health. The first symptoms (fever, chills) occurred on 2 July and she was admitted to a general hospital on 5 July. Rapid clinical deterioration with liver failure and severe haemorrhage occurred on 7 July and she was transferred to another University Medical Center, placed in quarantine, and medical care was provided. Approximately 100 close contacts of this woman closely monitored by a medical team. The patient finally died on July the 11th.

Chapter 2

PREPARING THE HEALTH CARE SYSTEM

Planning to prepare the health care system for a pandemic influenza or other disease outbreaks is difficult because of many, already mentioned, uncertainties. Indeed, strikingly little clinical and epidemiological information is known from the human cases of avian influenza to date [83], although most information points at a sepsis-like pattern with a pro-inflammatory cytokine storm [10]. Many of the characteristics relevant for the planning, such as disease attack rate, hospital and intensive care (ICU) admission rate, mechanical ventilation rate, hospital and ICU length of stay and mortality can be factored in only after the new virus has emerged [81]. Almost all assumptions in published models have drawn on knowledge from the past twentieth century pandemics [84-86].

The traditional public health approach to yearly seasonal influenza epidemics has three components: (1) vaccination of high-risk populations, including Health Care Workers (HCWs); (2) chemoprophylaxis of exposed high-risk populations; and (3) treatment of populations at high risk for complications from influenza. However, the public health response to an influenza pandemic is very different. First, it is unlikely that any (or enough) vaccine will be available quickly enough to prevent significant morbidity and mortality. Second, the population at high risk for complications is greater then historically expected [74]. Finally, it is unlikely that an influenza pandemic will be contained among health care workers even if excellent infection control practices are followed. The protection of health care workers and the public at large will depend more on available antiviral drugs for chemoprophylaxis and treatment than on vaccination, although some beneficial effect of vaccination might be expected [74].

Chapter 3

IMPACT OF AVIAN INFLUENZA IN THE NETHERLANDS

In case an influenza pandemic will reach Europe and the Netherlands, health care systems would have to play an essential role in controlling the effects of the disease for the general public. The impact of an influenza pandemic in the Netherlands on number of patients, number of general practitioners consults, number of hospital admissions and in hospital mortality is presented in table 1.

Data on population ($\approx$16.5 million) and age distribution were obtained from publicly available sources and numbers of the impact of a pandemic influenza on health care services were adopted from the National Institute for Public Health and the Environment (RIVM) to construct Table 1 [78,87]. The models assume a gross attack rate of 30%, and an in-hospital mortality of approximately 40% [78,87]. Only 2% of all patients seeking general practitioners' consultation are admitted to a hospital, consisting of 0.3% of all patients falling ill. The Dutch health care services constitute eight tertiary medical centers and ten trauma centers and 86 general hospitals in a total of 122 locations, not including nursing homes, hospices etc.

Table 1. Impact of Avian Influenza in the Netherlands

30% Attack Rate *					
Week No.	Days	No. Patients	General Practitioners consultations	No. of Hosp. Adm.	In-hospital Mortality
0	1 - 7	0	0	0	0
1	8 - 14	989	99	0	0
2	15 - 21	44,226	4,848	99	0
3	22 - 28	1,374,771	156,028	2,968	792
4	29 - 35	3,272,441	421,188	9,201	3,958
5	36 - 42	244,382	34,827	890	693
6	43 - 49	5,442	792	0	0
7	50 - 56	99	0	0	0
8	57 - 63	0	0	0	0
9	64 - 70	0	0	0	0
Total		4,942,350	617,781	13,159	5,442

* 30% attack rate, pandemic period 9 weeks; Week No. = week number; Days = days after onset of the pandemic; No. Patients = number of patients with ILI; General Practitioners consultations = number of GP consultations; No. of Hosp. Adm.; number of hospital admissions; In-hospital Mortality= number of deaths in hospital.

Chapter 4

HOSPITAL CAPACITY

Surge capacity of hospital resources is typically limited [79]. Hospital and intensive care beds will pose to be one of the critical and scarce resources if large numbers of influenza like illness (ILI) patients need to be admitted. The Dutch general hospitals own a total of 44,784 hospital beds while the eight tertiary medical centres contain 6,624 hospital beds. This leads to 27 general hospital beds per 10,000 inhabitants and 4 tertiary hospital beds per 10,000 inhabitants. In contrast, in Africa the number of general hospital beds per 10,000 inhabitants ranges between 2 and 14 (census 2005). In the Americas (North and South America) the number of general hospitals beds ranges from 67 (Barbados and United States of America) per 10,000 inhabitants to 7 hospital beds per 10,000 (Guatemala).

Chapter 5

INTENSIVE CARE UNIT CAPACITY

ICU beds are an integral part of public health care in The Netherlands [88]. Level 1-3 ICU's provide services for critically ill patients; Level 1 provides provisional care (<24-48h) for patients with shock and / or respiratory failure and has; with limited capacity and limited level of training of staff; Levels 2-3 have all facilities available for patients with multiple organ dysfunction, and are able to provide the full range of support; these units are fully staffed with ICU nursing and medical staff around the clock. Many hospitals also have designated intensive care areas for certain specialities of medicine (e.g. burn units, neurosurgery units, thoracic surgery), as dictated by the needs and available resources of each hospital [89-92]. After adjustment for severity of illness, demographic variables, and characteristics of the ICUs (including staffing by intensive care physicians), higher ICU volume is significantly associated with lower ICU and hospital mortality rates [90-93]. Typically, patient to nurse ratio is what determines the level of care [94-96]. A ratio of 2 patients to 1 nurse is recommended for a medical ICU. This is unlike the ratio of 4:1 or 5:1 ratio on the medical floors. In the United Kingdom, intensive care medicine is an extremely specialized area. In the United States, up to 20% of hospital beds can be labelled as intensive care beds, whereas in the United Kingdom intensive care usually will comprise only up to 2% of total beds. In the Netherlands this ratio is approximately similar to the United Kingdom. This high disparity is attributed to patients in the UK and the Netherlands who are admitted to an ICU tending to be only the most severely ill. Intensive Care is a expensive healthcare service and ICU beds are therefore a very scarce resource, even in most affluent countries [88]. ICU beds are indispensable in controlling the effects and reducing morbidity and mortality of a disease outbreak. It is assumed that the majority of all patients with Influenza Like Illness (ILI), admitted to a hospital, will require some form of mechanical ventilation available only in an ICU environment.

For hospital resources (i.e. availability of hospital and ICU beds), the mere number of expected ILI patients in an influenza pandemic will pose no strain on available resources. The strain comes from the time period an ILI patient occupies a hospital or ICU bed. On the basis of experience with patients admitted to the ICU with a diagnosis of pneumonia or sepsis (equivalent to patients with ILI requiring ICU admission) predictions will range from 8 to 15 days that patients with ILI will occupy a hospital or ICU bed. The number of admissions will be additive during an influenza pandemic and hence quickly drain away all available resources from public health services and hospitals.

Menon et al showed through a simulation study that critical care capacity in the United Kingdom would be overwhelmed even in case of a mild (AR <30%) influenza pandemic [86]. They predict a demand for critical care beds of 208% far exceeding the existing capacity. Anderson et al showed in a similar study in the Australasia region, that in a mild pandemic the number of hospital and intensive care beds would suffice [97]. They state also that if however, a worst case scenario would be anticipated in Australasia, there would be a shortfall of up to 228,993 bed days.

Chapter 6

WORKFORCE

In the Netherlands a major part of preparedness planning for a pandemic consists of maintaining essential public services, e.g., police, fire departments, army personnel, and healthcare workers (HCWs). HCWs will play a dominant role in containing and controlling disease outbreaks and caring for ILI patients. The recent SARS, Ebola and avian influenza outbreaks have placed these HCWs at disproportionate risks of serious morbidity and mortality from infection, and consequently it cannot be assumed that HCWs are willing to work normally even if they are able to do so despite professional obligations [98]. During the SARS outbreak of 2003, for instance, it was found that some HCWs were not willing to treat SARS patients [99,100]. Health care services contingency planning, and consequently patient care, would be improved with the possibility of predicting the factors that affect HCWs' willingness to work. Some barriers to willingness to work have already been identified, such as a high risk for self and family and care for sick family members [101-104]. In their survey among hospital staff in a university hospital, Ehrenstein et al found 28% of professionals (clinical and non-clinical) may abandon work in favor of protecting themselves, leaving 72% of hospital staff caring for patients with ILI [102]. Qureshi et al found HCWs in 47 health care facilities in New York City to be least *willing* to report for duty during a catastrophic disaster as SARS outbreak (48% willing to work) or a smallpox epidemic (61% willing to work) [103] In a survey in three health departments in Maryland, Balicer et al found that only 54% of clinical staff will be likely to report for duty during a pandemic, and they showed that clinical staff was more willing to work than non-clinical staff [105]. A recent study by Masterson et al among emergency department personnel showed a decrease in willingness to work of 42.7% if the disaster was a biological agent, leaving 57% of HCWs willing to work [106]. And finally, a survey from Alexander and Wynia under patient-care physicians extracted from the American Medical association Masterfile of all licensed physicians in the United States showed a narrow majority of 55% of agreement that physicians have an obligation to care for patients in epidemics even if doing so endangers the physicians' health [107].

Chapter 7

GENERAL PRACTITIONERS

In case of a pandemic influenza, general practitioners will be among the first HCWs finding themselves confronted with ILI patients. In the Netherlands there are approximately 7.100 general practitioners, leading to one general practitioner per 2.331 inhabitants. General practitioners will play also a predominant role in controlling pandemic influenza: T, they know the population they serve, they will perform first triage, and they will have to decide who among ILI patients will benefit from hospital admission and who will be left at home (either to recover or die). Hospitals will rely on general practitioners not to overload the hospitals with ILI patients preventing the hospitals to provide the best care to the most severe ILI patients.

Chapter 8

AGE DISTRIBUTION

As mentioned previously in this chapter, it is unknown which age groups will be most affected by an influenza pandemic. If the next influenza pandemic will be like the 1918–1919 strain there would be a high rate of mortality among patients between the ages of 15 and 35 years. To date, among the total number of reported avian influenza cases and deaths to the WHO, 50% were children (<19 yrs of age). In the Netherlands the age specific attack rates are 37.4% for age group 0-18 years, 28.6% for age group 19-64 and 23.1%for age group 65 years and older. These figures are comparable to the age distribution of reported cases to the WHO [78].

Specific attention to hospitalization of children is justified, the effect of using neuraminidase inhibitors to treat influenza in children is still uncertain and children have increased risk of bacterial pneumonia after ILI with increased risk of dying [25,72]. Also, until now pediatric HCWs are also underrepresented in national and local pandemic influenza preparedness planning [25,72,108].

The report by the Writing Committee of the WHO Consultation on Human Influenza shows a case fatality rate of 61% in total, especially among age group 10-19 years and a lower rate in age group 50 years and older which is markedly different from observations in earlier pandemics [22,30,37,109]. So far, it is assumed that age group 10 -19 years only makes up a small percentage of hospital admissions. One of the important questions is whether this age group is at particular risk worldwide or if it differs per region. In the Netherlands there are two million persons between 10 and 19 years (=12% of the total population, Europe 11.7%). For affluent countries, the economic ramifications of "loosing" the younger generation by to avian influenza might be even more dramatic then the pandemic itself because of an increasing older population. As mentioned previously, the majority of ILI patients admitted to a hospital would benefit from admission to an ICU environment. Miranda and Nap (2007) showed that age is not a contributing factor in a priori mortality [110] Although the younger population will probably be at increased risk and loosing a younger generation to pandemic influenza will pose an immense strain on the economic future, age discrimination has been forbidden in the USA since 1975 (the Age Discrimination Act). In the "Standard one – rooting out age discrimination", the British Department of Health states: "NHS services will be provided, regardless of age, on the basis of clinical need alone. Social care services will not use age in their eligibility criteria or policies, to restrict access to available services". Before these documents appeared, expressions of aggressive discrimination were not uncommon, such as: accepting the use of age as a criterion for rationing ICU beds, or the adoption of principles of justice to ensure the impartial distribution of scarce resources. It is recognized that age does matter regarding the outcome of illness in ICU patients. The importance of age concerns only the progressive and age-related reduction of the physiological reserve. From a clinical point of view, therefore, older patients may require specific attention, because earlier implementation of supportive interventions may be required, but age can not be a discriminating factor in triage and access to public health services or hospitals.

Chapter 9

UNDERLYING DISEASE AND CO-MORBIDITY

An additional complicating factor for health care services to date, as compared to the pandemics in the 20th century, is the increasing population with an underlying disease and/or co-morbidity. This high-risk proportion of the population suffers from consists of a number of diseases identified as contributors to influenza-related excess mortality. This includes Chronic Obstructive Pulmonary Disease (COPD), cancer, cerebral-vascular accident, chronic heart disease and diabetes mellitus [38,111]. The high-risk proportion of the population in The Netherlands is different in different age groups. In the age group below 18 years, this is 2.4%, in the age group between 19 and 64 years, 6.2%; and in the age group above 65 years, 35%. This high-risk population will place additional strain on already scarce health care services resources during an influenza pandemic.

Chapter 10

MITIGATION OF PANDEMIC INFLUENZA

Scenarios for worldwide pandemic containment or mitigation usually consist of four main factors: early containment, travel restrictions, vaccination, and therapeutic and prophylactic use of anti-viral drugs.

In an emerging pandemic, when the causative agent (probably, virus) is known, the production and deployment of adequate vaccine supplies would require a time period in the order of six to eight months [112]. Global travel limitations, but also quarantine, early isolation of infectious individuals, school and workplace closures are considered non-pharmaceutical interventions aimed at containing the virus spread within populations and are recommended by the WHO. However, but a number of these interventions would be unfeasible since they are regarded as economically too disruptive [11,15,82,113-115]. It has also been shown that even drastic travel limitations delay the pandemic evolution by only a few weeks, with almost no impact on morbidity [84]. The international community would therefore have to rely initially on anti-viral drugs, mainly the neuraminidase inhibitor drugs oseltamivir and zanamivir, which represent a viable response measure to a pandemic in the absence of a vaccine and of other feasible interventions [116]. The WHO has a stockpile of oseltamivir to use in early cases of human-to-human transmissions of a potential pandemic virus to attempt to slow the outbreak and create more time for vaccine production and other preparations. However, the unknowns regarding a potential pandemic virus, including how quickly the virus spreads, the efficacy of the drugs, and the rate of acquisition of drug resistance by the virus make it difficult to predict how useful a drug stockpiling strategy would be [67,74,117-119].

Chapter 11

CONTAINMENT MEASURES FOR PANDEMIC INFLUENZA

The endemic nature of current avian influenza among domestic birds and their close co-existence with humans in rural areas of Asia makes this part of the world a likely epicentre for an avian influenza pandemic. Ferguson et al and Longini et al used computer modelling to simulate what may happen if avian influenza were to start being transmitted efficiently between people in Southeast Asia [11,113]. Both groups showed that a carefully selected and orchestrated combination of public health measures could potentially stop the spread of an avian influenza pandemic if implemented soon after the first cases appear. The proposed strategies include an international stockpile of antiviral drugs, treating infected individuals and everyone in their social networks, closure of schools and workplaces, vaccination (even with a low-efficacy vaccine) of half the population before the start of a pandemic, and quarantine measures. Targeted anti-viral treatment is an important component of all strategies and increasing public health measures needed to be increased when the virus becomes more contagious. While the researchers acknowledged that implementing such a combination of approaches was challenging because it required a coordinated international response, the models show that containing an avian influenza pandemic at its source is theoretically feasible.

To successfully contain and control an avian influenza pandemic, global, national and local strategies are needed. National strategies need multi-pronged approaches and involve source surveillance and control, adequate national stockpiles of antivirals, timely production of influenza vaccines when feasible and healthcare system readiness. When the pandemic influenza virus becomes easily transmissible from human to human, the earlier this fact is known, the more time there will be to gather and deploy available public health resources. Currently, the WHO, United Nations and other international agencies are trying to contain the H5N1 epidemic among poultry flocks in Asia and have set up monitoring systems to detect new outbreaks (especially human-to-human cases) early. Recently an internet-based alarm system model was published that might help in the early detection of such a pandemic [120]. Recent models built on data from the 1918 flu pandemic predict that 50 million-80 million people could die and that the overwhelming majority of deaths are likely to occur in the developing countries. After six months the development of a protective vaccine will be finished and mass production will start. Total global capacity for this vaccine manufacture in the first 12 months is estimated at only 500 million doses, which will definitely not suffice. Moreover production faces many constraints: The vaccine is cultured in eggs, and this is a time consuming process which cannot be speeded up [121]. Therefore alternative sources of virus culture cells are being investigated [122-125]. With avian influenza affecting poultry and eggs, the egg supply required for vaccine production may itself be disrupted. Intellectual property rights and liability from adverse effects from vaccines are other issues that impede manufacturers from increasing vaccine production. It should also be noted that if the influenza pandemic strain turns out not to be the H5N1 variety, then the stockpiled vaccines would probably be useless and wasted. Deciding whom to vaccinate is another challenge. Influenza vaccination against seasonal influenza is recommended for the elderly and those with underlying medical conditions because they are at higher risk for hospitalization and death if they become infected with influenza. Some critics have argued that younger and healthier individuals should be given priority because they are more mobile than older, less healthy people and are therefore more likely to contract and spread pandemic influenza. Another factor in favour of giving priority to younger people is that the seasonal influenza vaccine produces a weaker immune response in the elderly, so that their contribution to herd immunity is also less. Also, if the influenza pandemic has the same characteristics as the 1918–1919 pandemic, then the young and healthy are at higher risk of death. Even if supplies were adequate for all age groups, mass immunization for a potential pandemic still has its risks. In 1976, four US soldiers developed swine flu in an army camp and there was concern that it could become a pandemic like the 1918 Spanish flu [126]. Although some health officials expressed doubts about the likelihood of an epidemic, the government initiated a mass inoculation programme for the entire US population. After hundreds of people receiving the vaccine came down with Guillain-Barré syndrome, the

US government terminated the campaign and sued the manufacturers in court. Recently the WHO announced plans to stockpile H5 influenza vaccine and create a policy framework for vaccine allocation and recommendations for its use [127]. Several recent developments in H5 vaccines have made this stockpile feasible: the development of H5N1 vaccines with adjuvants that reduce the required dose as much as fourfold and the finding that adjuvant-enhanced vaccines may provide cross-protection against strains that have undergone up to seven years of genetic drift [128,129].

The economic cost of an avian pandemic to all countries would be immense and, if allowed to last for months, become exponential [130,131]. Early detection and control of an influenza pandemic will require a coordinated international response. The response to the influenza threat would need an integrated cross-sector approach, bringing together animal and human health, areas of rural development and agriculture, economics, finance and planning. Partnerships are needed at international, national and local levels. Next, there is certainly a priority on curbing the disease "at source" in the agricultural sector, thereby reducing the probability of a human epidemic. International resources are also needed for surveillance on avian influenza outbreaks and human-to human transmission. Avian influenza is becoming endemic in parts of East Asia and will require a long effort to suppress it. Meanwhile, a human pandemic may still emerge from a different strain of flu virus. Thus it makes sense for the international community to undertake broader long-term measures to strengthen the institutional, regulatory and technical capacity of the animal health, human health and other relevant sectors. While country-level preparedness and leadership is essential for success, it must be backed by global resources. Even though the benefits of containing a pandemic are overwhelming, individual governments may still be daunted by the social, political and economic costs of various policy measures. Affluent countries need to support less affluent regions in the fight against an influenza pandemic. The Global Outbreak Alert & Response Network (GOARN), a technical collaboration of existing institutions and networks that pool human and technical resources for the rapid identification, confirmation and response to disease outbreaks, is one such international body that supports global preparedness against avian influenza. However, for such an organization to succeed, open communication and international cooperation is essential. There is a need to share information rapidly with experts, policymakers on international, national and local levels.

Chapter 12

HEALTHCARE SYSTEM READINESS

Every country's healthcare system would be stretched to the limit in the event of an influenza pandemic or any other disease outbreak. In all proposed and possible control and containment measures for pandemic influenza, a huge strain is placed on the surge capacity of public health services. The ability of healthcare facilities to maintain strict infection control measures would be challenged and the surge in health manpower and facility need would be acutely felt among healthcare workers. Hospitals will play a key role in regional and local preparedness planning. In order for this to work, cooperation needs to be established between all partners in health care delivery (e.g. general practitioners, hospitals, nursing homes, hospices etc.) and in case of a pandemic, previous competition between hospitals should immediately be stopped and managers should change gears to allow open communication and sharing of vital information. Preparedness planning for health services – both health services and hospitals – is a process that involves two major aspects: internal (business) and external (environment) preparation.

Chapter 13

INTERNAL PREPARATION

Besides their dedication to the welfare of the population they serve, hospitals and other public health services are also a business in their own right, with all necessary infrastructures (e.g. water, power, ever increasing dependence on information technology services, waste disposal, cleaning services etc.). For example, in March 2008 the UMCG was confronted with a breach in the main water supply serving the entire city of Groningen. A hospital, specifically hospitals in the size of the UMCG with 1,300 hospital beds, consumes 50 to 60 cubic meters of water an hour during normal production days, and 100 to 120 cubic meters of water an hour during peak hours. For problems like this, the UMCG holds two water tanks in the basement containing a total of 180 cubic meters of water. The crisis management team made some rigorous decisions in order to save as much water for patient care as possible, which is critical to fulfill their primary purpose. Because the breach occurred on a Monday morning, all personnel were screened at the front door, and subsequently, non-essential personnel were sent home. The trauma helicopter was grounded on the flight deck on top of the roof of the hospital, because no water in case of fire after an accident was available and all sprinklers were cut off from water, changing to alternate sources of fire fighting. All outpatients' clinics, including the dialysis unit, were closed and most of the toilets were shut by security officers. If patients had to be washed, special washing clothes were used, containing soap and alcohol, preventing the use of water. The water company provided trucks with water tanks to replenishing the draining basement water tanks. The water breach was solved after 48 hours and quality was back to the drinking water levels. The evaluation of this internal "disaster" contained a number of critical functions which needed additional attention. For example, the basic water supply of the hospital was increased, and several departments and functions, previously not denoted as critical, were given a higher priority (e.g. dialysis outpatient clinic, pharmacy, blood bank and diagnostic laboratories) and back-up personnel and a back-up crisis management team were formed because the disaster stretched over a number of days, greatly decreasing the ability of the crisis management team to perform and make critical decisions. Another important piece of advice was to develop of a business continuity plan to ensure the critical functions of the hospital during disasters including a disease outbreak.

Chapter 14

BUSINESS CONTINUITY

Business continuity (planning) is the creation and validation of a practiced logistical plan for how an organization will recover and partially or completely restore interrupted critical (urgent) functions within a predetermined time after a disaster or extended disruption. The logistical plan is called a business continuity plan (BCP). In plain language, a business continuity plan is a standard operating procedure describing how to continue daily business in the event of a disaster and how to be back in business after the disaster has subsided. Incidents include local incidents like building fires, regional incidents like earthquakes, or national or international incidents like pandemic influenza. The BCP may be a part of an organizational learning effort that helps reduce operational risk. This process may be integrated with corporate risk management practices. Business continuity planning methodology is scalable for an organization of any size and complexity. Even though the methodology has roots in regulated industries, any type of organization may create a BCP. Evidence that firms do not invest enough time and resources into BCP preparations are evident in disaster survival statistics. For example, fires permanently close 44% of the business affected [132]. The need for zero downtime of critical processes is growing, emphasizing the need for prevention, not recovery, to be given more emphasis. This requires a fundamental shift in the traditional approach to business continuity. Under this new paradigm business continuity truly becomes a management discipline – managing the mission-critical business processes to ensure continuous availability. In the 1993 World Trade Centre bombing, 150 businesses of a total of 350 affected failed to survive the event. Conversely, the firms affected by the Sept. 11 attacks with well-developed and tested business continuity plans were back in business within days. Business continuity must bring all business protection issues under one umbrella, ensuring effective oversight of all mission critical processes, giving transparent insight into all areas of the organization and allowing effective continuity management. BCP sits alongside crisis management and disaster recovery planning and is a part of an organization's overall risk management. The analysis phase in the development of BCP consists of an impact analysis, threat analysis, and impact scenarios with the resulting BCP plan requirements. An impact analysis results in the differentiation between critical (urgent) and non-critical (non-urgent) organization functions/ activities. A function may be considered critical if the implications to the organization resulting from a disturbance or disaster are regarded as unacceptable. A function may also be considered critical if dictated by law. After defining recovery requirements, documenting potential threats is recommended to detail a specific disaster's unique recovery steps. Some common defined threats include the following; disease, earthquake, fire, flood, cyber attack, hurricane, utility outage and terrorism. All threats in the examples above share a common impact: the potential of damage to organizational infrastructure - except one (disease). The impact of diseases can be regarded as purely human, and may be alleviated with technical and business solutions. However, if the humans behind these recovery plans are also affected by the disease, then the process can fall down. During the 2002-2003 SARS outbreak, some organizations grouped staff into separate teams, and rotated the teams between the primary (with infected patients) and secondary work sites, with a rotation frequency equal to the incubation period of the disease. The organizations also banned face-to-face contact between opposing team members during business and non-business hours. With such a split, organizations increased their resiliency against the threat of government-ordered quarantine measures if one person in a team contracted or was exposed to the disease. After defining potential threats, documenting the impact scenarios that form the basis of the business recovery plan is recommended. In general, planning for the most wide-reaching disaster or disturbance is preferable to planning for a smaller scale problem, as almost all smaller scale problems are partial elements of larger disasters. After the completion of the analysis phase, the business and technical requirements are documented in order to commence an implementation phase for business continuity and a solution phase. The solution phase determines the crisis management command structure. The nature of emergency management depends on local economic and social conditions. Experts have long noted that the cycle of emergency management must include long-term work on infrastructure, public awareness, and even human justice issues. This is particularly important in developing nations. The process of emergency management involves four phases: *mitigation, preparedness, response,* and *recovery*. Mitigation efforts attempt to prevent hazards developing into disasters or to reduce the effects of disasters when they occur. The mitigation phase differs from the other phases because it focuses on long-term measures for eliminating or reducing risk. The implementation of mitigation strategies can be considered a part of the recovery process if applied after a disaster occurs. Mitigative measures can be structural or non-structural. Structural measures use technological solutions, like flood levees. Non-structural measures include legislation, land-use planning (e.g. the designation of nonessential land like parks to be used as flood zones), and insurance. Mitigation is the most cost-efficient method for reducing the impact of hazards; however it is not always suitable. Some structural mitigation measures may have adverse effects on the ecosystem. A precursor activity to the mitigation is the identification of risks or risk management. Physical risk assessment refers to the process of identifying and evaluating hazards. The hazard-specific risk combines both the probability and the level of impact of a specific hazard, the higher the risk, the more urgent that the hazard specific vulnerabilities are targeted by mitigation and preparedness efforts. However, if there is no vulnerability there will be no risk, e.g.such as when earthquakes occurring in a desert where nobody lives. In the *preparedness phase*, emergency managers develop plans of action for when the disaster strikes. Common preparedness measures include: communication plans with easily understandable terminology and methods; proper maintenance and training of emergency services, including mass human resources such as community emergency response teams; development and exercise of emergency population warning methods combined with emergency shelters and evacuation plans; stockpiling, inventory, and maintaining disaster supplies and equipment; and developing organizations of trained volunteers among civilian populations (professional emergency workers are rapidly overwhelmed in mass emergencies. Trained, organized and responsible volunteers are extremely valuable). Another aspect of preparedness is casualty prediction, the study of how many deaths or injuries to expect for a given kind of event. This gives planners an idea of what resources need to be in place to respond to a particular kind of event. The *response phase* includes the mobilization of the necessary emergency services and first responders in the disaster area. This is likely to include a first wave of core emergency services, such as fire-fighters, police and ambulance crews. They may be supported by a number of secondary emergency services, such as specialist rescue teams. A well rehearsed emergency plan developed as part of the preparedness phase enables efficient coordination of rescue. The response phase of an emergency may commence with search and rescue but in all cases the focus will quickly turn to fulfilling the basic humanitarian needs of the affected population. Assistance may be provided by national or international agencies and organisations. Effective coordination of disaster assistance is often crucial, particularly when many organisations respond and local emergency management agency capacity has been exceeded by the demand or diminished by the disaster itself. The aim of the *recovery phase* is to restore the affected area to its previous state. It differs from the response phase in its focus; recovery efforts are concerned with issues and decisions that must be made after immediate needs are addressed. Recovery efforts are primarily concerned with actions that involve rebuilding destroyed property, re-employment, and the repair of other essential infrastructure. An important aspect of effective recovery efforts is taking advantage of a 'window of opportunity' for the implementation of mitigative measures that might otherwise be unpopular. Citizens of the affected area are more likely to accept more mitigative changes when a recent disaster is in fresh memory. Personal mitigation is mainly about knowing and avoiding unnecessary risks. This includes an assessment of possible risks to personal/family health and to personal property. Mitigation involves structural and non-structural measures taken to limit the impact of disasters (e.g. mitigation activities, which are aimed at preventing a disaster from occurring, personal preparedness focuses on preparing equipment and procedures for use when a disaster occurs, i.e. planning). Preparedness measures can take many forms including the construction of shelters, installation of warning devices, creation of back-up life-line services (e.g. power, water, sewage), and rehearsing evacuation plans. The recovery phase starts after the immediate threat to human life has subsided. In the past, the field of emergency management has been populated mostly by people with a military or first responder background. Currently, the population in the field has become more diverse, with many experts coming from a variety of backgrounds and having no military or first responder history at all.

Chapter 15

EXTERNAL PREPARATION

Besides internal preparation for disturbances and disasters, hospitals also need external preparation. Under Dutch law, the UMCG, as a trauma center and regional coordinating centre, would plays an important role in the case of an (avian) influenza pandemic [133]. Although hospitals are in constant competition with other hospitals, for patients and for governmental funding, in case of a disease outbreak it is imperative that hospitals, general practitioners, hospices and nursing homes share information, usually regarded as confidential, such as that regarding number of hospital and intensive care beds, occupancy ratios, number of health care workers etc. Because the surge capacity of all health care services is limited, strict information sharing and clear triage rules are vital to assure optimum care for those patients who stand to benefit the most. With regional and municipal health authorities, general practitioners, and representatives of all hospitals in the Northern region, information and training courses were held for pandemic influenza, emphasizing the need to enhance collaboration and communication in July 2006 and emphasizing the concept of fair share of among all partners in health care. The threat of a global disease outbreak in the future with internal and external preparation and co-dependencies between all public health services, forces hospital managers to change their management of the hospital and direct attention towards health care as a regional entity instead of a local business. This demands preparation in "peace time" is necessary to be able to cope with the increased demand during "war time".

Very limited literature is available that discusses the consequences of the failure to prepare in health care. The influenza pandemic of 1918 was the source of much fear in citizens around the world. Further inflaming that fear was the fact that governments and health officials were downplaying the influenza. While the panic from WWI was dwindling, governments attempted to keep morale up by spreading lies and dismissing the influenza. On Sept. 11, 1918, Washington officials reported that the Spanish Influenza had arrived in the city. The following day, roughly thirteen 13 million men across the country lined up to register for the war draft, providing the influenza with an efficient way to spread. However, the influenza had little impact upon institutions and organizations. While medical scientists rapidly attempted to discover a cure or vaccine, there were virtually no changes in the government or in corporations. Consequently, an estimated one third of the world's population (or ≈500 million persons) was infected and had clinically apparent illness [134,135].

During the global SARS outbreak of 2003, in Toronto, Canada, 225 residents met the case definition of SARS, and all but 3 travel-related cases were linked to the index patient, from Hong Kong. SARS spread to 11 (58 percent) of Toronto's acute care hospitals. Unrecognized SARS among in-patients with underlying illness caused resurgence, or a second phase, of the outbreak, which was finally controlled through active surveillance of hospitalized patients, not in place initially. In response to the control measures of Toronto Public Health, the number of persons who were exposed to SARS in non-hospital and non-household settings dropped from 20 persons before the control measures were instituted to 0 after the measures were instituted. The number of patients who were exposed while in a hospital ward rose from 25 patients to 68 patients, and the number exposed while in the intensive care unit dropped from 13 patients to 0 patients [136]. Community spread (the length of the chains of transmission outside hospital settings) was significantly reduced after installment of control measures. The transmission of SARS in Toronto was limited primarily to hospitals and to households that had had contact with patients. During an outbreak, active in-hospital surveillance for SARS-like illnesses and heightened infection-control measures are essential. These measures were not in place before the onset of SARS and although it is difficult to estimate the excess human suffering, it can be postulated that this second wave of SARS could (partially) have been prevented [137].

Lipshitz (1994) shows that real-world decision making reveals three types of, mutually exclusive, fundamentally different decision making processes: *consequential choice* (the concurrent choice between options with certain, risky or uncertain outcomes), *matching* (matching of actions to situations or solutions to problems, mostly on the basis of past experience, intuitions, habits and training as well as personal values at the individual level; and standard operating procedures, norms and professional and ideological doctrines at the group and organizational level) and *reassessment* (describes failures of critical reassement, it is decision making after the decision has already been made) [138]. The basic conclusion is that real-world decisions are embedded in networks of paradigmatic assumptions of which decision makers may or may not be aware. Lipshitz also shows that decision makers are more likely to meet their objectives if they employ a mindful decision process (being totally present in the here and now and perceiving things as they are without making additional assumptions) [139]. The norms that facilitate mindful decision making are: inquiry (persisting in investigation until full understanding is achieved), integrity (collecting and providing information regardless of its implications), transparency (exposing one's thoughts and actions to others) and issue orientation (focusing on the relevance of information to the issues regardless of the social standing or rank of the recipient or the source) [140]. Lipshitz showed that the Israel Defence Force (I.D.F.) decision making process in the Second Lebanon War was hampered by failing to reflect critically on close held assumptions, mindless awareness of actual situations, misinterpreted communication and closely relying on standard operating procedures on individual, group and organizational level. The second Lebanon War lasted 34 days between July 12 and August 14, 2006. This period, in which events repeatedly seemed to elude planners' designs and intentions, partly or largely because calculated risks turned out, in retrospect, to have been risky calculations, can be summarized as follows;

On July 12 a Hezbollah unit attacks an I.D.F. patrol and kidnaps two soldiers. Concurrently it launches a diversionary rocket attack on civilian settlements along the entire length of Israel's border with Lebanon. A tank which crosses the border in pursuit of the kidnappers hits a huge roadside charge. The tank is destroyed and its crew of four is killed. Altogether, the I.D.F. suffers eight dead soldiers in the skirmishes that follow the kidnapping incident. Contrary to Nasrallah's (Hezbollah's charismatic leader) intentions, the I.D.F.'s Chief of Staff, Israel's government, and Israeli public opinion do not interpret the incident as a Hezbollah attempt to force Israel to bargain and free Hezbollah fighters that it holds as prisoners. Rather, the kidnapping is perceived as a strategic threat to further weaken Israel's deterring power which had suffered a blow from a successful Hamas kidnapping operation in the Gaza Strip. After first attempting to interdict the kidnapper's routes back north, the I.D.F. responds on July13 with an extensive air campaign. Chief of Staff Halutz is reluctantly forced to replace the I.D.F.'s air-based strategy by a land-based strategy to which its reserve units, in particular, were ill prepared. The results were recurrent equipment shortages, frequently mixed outcomes of the ground force's clashes with Hezbollah units, and disgruntled soldiers and officers who explicitly criticized the I.D.F.'s high command and the government for taking ill advised decisions, and for sending poorly trained and under equipped units to war throughout southern Lebanon. Hezbollah's long-range rockets (capable of reaching Tel Aviv) are destroyed, and civilian installations suspected of serving as Hezbollah supply routes (e.g., Beirut's International Airport and the Beirut–Damascus highway) also suffer damages. A general sea and air blockade is imposed later on. As the war escalates life in northern Israel becomes intolerable for civilians. Although the number of casualties is low, they live in fear, and spend long time periods in inadequate underground shelters. The I.D.F.'s air campaign causes much costlier human and material losses. Nevertheless, it fails to stop the intermittent firing of medium and short range rockets. On October 1st the I.D.F. has withdrawn all its forces from Lebanon with two minor exceptions where the exact location of the international border is disputed. Hezbollah has moved its units back and does not maintain overt presence along the Israel-Lebanon Border. In contradiction to UN Security Council Resolution 1701 which ended the war, both the Lebanese government and UNIFIL (the UN's observers force in Lebanon) have explicitly stated that they will not disarm Hezbollah. The situation of the two I.D.F. soldiers and the Hezbollah prisoners, on whose behalf they were kidnapped, was not changed. The I.D.F. failed, at least in part, because the decision making processes that guided its planning and operations suffered from mindless awareness of the situation on the ground and uncritical adherence to its plans, assumptions, and paradigms.

Lipshitz argues that decision making consists of four basic rules: be *mindful* (e.g. of the effectiveness or ineffectiveness of the methods to be chosen to achieve an objective); and *critical* (e.g. of the underlying assumptions of the methods); use *profound simplicity* and *common sense* as guiding principles when no theory or doctrine is available. In order for hospital management to prepare for their changing role in the continuation of public health and to ensure optimal decision making during disease outbreaks, evidence based management, incorporating all above mentioned items, can proof to be an invaluable tool.

Chapter 16

EVIDENCE-BASED MANAGEMENT

As mentioned before, structured planning and preparation for disease outbreaks is not yet common ground for most health services, including hospitals and large tertiary referral centres. This may be difficult in affluent countries but obviously this is even more difficult in less affluent countries. It demands commitment from health care services ranging from the level of individual health care workers to government level to provide sufficient strategic decision making and financial resources for internal and external preparedness. It also demands a change in culture and focus, and communication of hospital management including the recognition of the ethical impact disease outbreaks have on clinicians and nurses who have to make day to day end of life decisions, specifically when resources are scarce.

The importance of evidence-based medicine (EBM) ("the conscientious, explicit and judicious use of current best evidence in making decisions about the care of individual patients) and modelling in preparing for disease outbreaks has to be encompassed by evidence-based management of the entire health care system. It requires the integration of (medical) content and context in which medical care has to be delivered. This is where evidence-based management will provide an essential role. Evidence-Based Management (EBMgt) enhances the overall quality of organizational decisions and practices through deliberative use of relevant and best available scientific evidence, which includes making use of disease outbreaks models and knowledge about surge capacity on regional, national and international level. To successfully implement EBMgt health care, managers should:

1 Face the hard facts, and build a culture in which personnel and management are encouraged to tell the truth, even if it is unpleasant;
2 Be committed to "fact based" decision making -- which means being committed to getting the best evidence and using it to guide actions [141];
3 Treat their organization as an unfinished prototype -- encourage experimentation and learning by doing;
4 Look for the risks and drawbacks in what advisors recommend -- even the best medicine has side effects;
5 Avoid basing decisions on untested but strongly held beliefs, what you have done in the past, or on uncritical "benchmarking" of what "successful" organizations do [141,142].

Like its counterparts in medicine [143] and education [144], the judgments EBMgt entails also consider the circumstances (context) and ethical concerns managerial decisions involve. In contrast to medicine and education, EBMgt today is only hypothetical. Contemporary managers and management educators make limited use of the vast behavioral science evidence base relevant to effective management practice [142,145-147]. Efforts to promote EBMgt face greater challenges than have other evidence-based initiatives. Unlike medicine, nursing, education, and law enforcement, "management" is not a profession. There are no established legal or cultural requirements regarding education or knowledge for an individual to become a manager. Managers have diverse disciplinary backgrounds. No formal body of shared knowledge characterizes managers, making it unlikely that peer pressure will be exerted to promote use of evidence by any manager who refuses to do so. Little shared language or terminology exists, making it difficult for managers to hold discussions of evidence or evidence-based practices [145,146]. For this reason, the adoption of evidence-based practices is likely to be organization-specific, where leaders take the initiative to build an evidence based culture [142]. Practices and evidence-based organizational culture include systematic accumulation and analysis of data gathered on the organization and its functioning, problem-based reading and discussion of research summaries by managers and staff, and the making of organizational decisions informed by both best available research and organizational information. Organizations successfully pursuing evidence-based management typically go through cycles of experimentation and redesign of their practices to create an evidence-based culture consistent with their values and mission.

To promote and adopt EBMgt, managers have identified four key strategies:

1 Recognize and respond to the growing demand for accountability as a strategic issue. Today, effective decision-making about highly scrutinized issues, such as a merger, as well as decisions on less visible but important issues, such as implementing components of the chronic care model, recruiting and retaining personnel, and implementing information technology, have strategic importance. Leaders should make it clear that their decisions are based on the best evidence available—that is, they have anticipated the consequences of their decisions, demonstrated good stewardship of resources and acted to ensure their organization's viability by using the best information available to improve performance;
2 Establish organizational structures and processes for knowledge transfer. Knowledge management involves identifying, creating, representing and distributing knowledge for reuse, awareness and learning across the organization. Organizations can assign this responsibility to individuals or teams within the organization, which should keep the knowledge management environment "live" through frequent communication with managers, physicians, nurses and others;
3 Build a questioning organizational culture. By creating and sustaining a "questioning" culture, the use of EBMgt will follow. Strategies for building a questioning culture include encouraging managers to challenge the evidence base for important decisions, having managers participate in research "rounds" or journal clubs, and comparing the organization's performance with research findings from other organizations;
4 Build organizational research capabilities. Organizations need to train managers in evidence-informed decision-making and establish "linkage and exchange" relationships with universities, research centres, and consulting firms and other knowledge brokers, and individual researchers. Another strategy for building research capabilities is to conduct in-house research on important issues, before and after these decisions are made. Managers who conduct their own studies, focus groups or market assessments have more knowledge and are more supportive of EBMgt. Successful EBMgt requires continual leadership by boards, executives, clinical staff and

managers (organizational, group and individual level). In particular, board and executive leadership must focus attention on the intersection of the quality, efficiency and access of EBMgt [148].

Two components are necessary to improve the quality of medical care: advances in evidence-based medicine (EBM), which identifies the clinical practices leading to better care, i.e., the *content* of providing care, and knowledge of how to put this content into routine practice and advances in EBMgt, which identifies the organizational strategies, structures, and change management practices that enable physicians and other health care professionals to provide evidence-based care, i.e., the *context* of providing care. Until both components are in place – identifying the best content (EBM) and applying it within effective organizational contexts (EBMgt) - consistent, sustainable improvement in the quality of care is unlikely to occur. Ensuring the delivery of high quality care, also during disease outbreaks, requires integration of knowledge from EBM and EBMgt. The content of what should be done, e.g., evidence on which drug, medical device, procedure, or treatment plan is most likely to improve patient outcomes needs to take into account the organizational and community context in which the care is delivered. EBMgt focuses on the underlying organizational issues that influence how care is delivered. The evidence base comes largely from the social and behavioral sciences, human factors engineering, and the field of health services research. In addition EBMgt uses observational data and approaches such as the plan-do-study-act (PDSA) quality improvement method for making small scale changes to improve care [149].

To understand the value of using EBM and EBMgt together, consider the treatment of patients with acute coronary syndromes (ACS). Evidence-based guidelines recommend that symptomatic patients presenting in the emergency department (ED) receive immediate evaluation, in an effort to decrease the time between the onset of symptoms and the initiation of treatment. In practice, not all patients at risk for an ACS receive prompt evaluation or treatment because of factors that can vary across EDs, e.g., limited space creating triage bottlenecks. A number of hospitals, however, reduced its door-to-balloon time for patients with acute myocardial infarctions (AMI) after reviewing the existing management research on workflow processes and drawing upon case studies from similar hospitals on ways to initiate electrocardiograms faster in symptomatic patients [150]. These hospitals were able to use EBMgt knowledge to help put EBM into practice.

Within both EBM and EBMgt, there are substantial, similar barriers to evidence use: time pressures, perceived threats to autonomy, the preference for "colloquial" knowledge based on individual experiences, difficulty in accessing the evidence base, difficulty of differentiating useful and accurate evidence from the inaccurate or inapplicable, and lack of resources [147,151,152]. Integrating the two bodies of knowledge also requires practitioners who are aware of and able to draw upon evidence from the two areas [153,154]. Few physicians read management studies; -few managers read clinical studies; -and few persons read all relevant studies within their own field.

Chapter 17

EVIDENCE FROM FOCUSED MODELLING: A CASE STUDY FROM THE NETHERLANDS

In preparing public health services for disease outbreaks, it is necessary to join content and context through EBM and EBMgt, to ensure business continuity, both internally as well as for external preparation. Management of public health services in general and hospitals specifically must be aware of all information about disease outbreaks, individual physicians should be more "community based, instead of community placed", so, well aware of the context (e.g. hospital, general practice, nursing home etc.) in which they can focus on the content (e.g. individual patient) [155].

Chapter 18

HEALTHCARE SYSTEM READINESS

As mentioned above, an influenza pandemic would cause intense human suffering, disruption of social systems, impose major economic losses and greatly burden health care services. To prepare health services for a disease outbreak, close communication and sharing of business information between all health services providers (e.g. HCWs, hospital management, nursing home management, general practitioners, medical schools, nursing schools, hospices etc) is essential. For public health services it is essential to provide the HCWs with the essential context to be able to focus on the content. In order to bring the messages above home to the reader, we present the results of a detailed analysis of preparedness planning modelling in the Netherlands that we have pursued.

With regional and municipal health authorities, general practitioners, and representatives of all hospitals in the Northern region of The Netherlands, training courses were held for information sharing, emphasizing the need to enhance collaboration and communication. During the training courses business continuity plans and models were presented showing the impact of an influenza pandemic on the Northern Region of The Netherlands [156-160]. It became apparent that increased hospitalization in combination with HCWs absenteeism will have substantial, but manageable impact on hospital and ICU bed occupancy in the models that were developed. The need for surge capacity of hospital resources depends more on the combination of excess hospital admissions and length of stay than the mere number of hospital admissions. The general opinion was that an influenza pandemic can be managed, even allowing for emergency care for non influenza-related acute cases, only when robust triage, decision rules and anti viral therapy are used. Without withdrawing or withholding life support to those deemed to have no realistic chance of survival, the system is bound to collapse, elaborating the mutual dependence of public health services and HCWs. With appropriate regional and local patient management adequate health care can be provided even during the peak of the pandemic.

Chapter 19

HOSPITAL AND INTENSIVE CARE UNIT CAPACITY

Insight in hospital and intensive care unit capacity is essential to understand the impact of an influenza pandemic on surge capacity. FluSurge 2.0 was used together with a computer model in an Excel file to calculate the impact of an influenza pandemic in The Netherlands on hospital admission, occupancy rate of all ICU [156,161]. Data on population in the Northern Region of The Netherlands (slightly over 1.7 million) and age distribution were obtained from publicly available sources. The age distribution in the Dutch population data were provided in blocks of five years, and we therefore converted these data to an even distribution to allow for calculations with the FluSurge program [86]. Data on total number of hospital beds, ICU beds and number of nurses and their full full-time equivalents were obtained from publicly available sources [162]. ICU capacity was also obtained from reports from hospital administrators during separate training sessions for pandemic influenza in May, 2006, organised by the Public Health authorities in the region. These data on reported ICU capacity were discussed during a semi-structured telephone interview with intensive care physicians in August, 2006. Based on these data estimation of regular bed capacity and maximal surge capacity was obtained. Numbers of the impact of a pandemic influenza on health care services were adopted from the National Institute for Public Health and the Environment (RIVM) [87,163]. The RIVM presented tables for 25% and 50% disease attack rates representing best and worst case scenarios. From these tables the 30% attack rate was calculated by linear transformation. A 30% attack rate is the most likely scenario according to the Centers for Disease Control and Prevention (CDC) and defined as the most likely scenario by the RIVM. Furthermore we calculated within the model the total number of patients on admission in the hospitals at each point in time during the pandemic. We defined the first day (day 0) as the moment WHO declares human to human transmission (phase IV or V in her current WHO phase of pandemic alert). The time each individual patient occupies a hospital or ICU bed (ranging from 8 to 15 days) was incorporated in the model based on experience with patients admitted to the ICU diagnosed with pneumonia or sepsis. Estimated mortality per patient was included in the model, reducing the number of admitted patients at any one time. Because the data of the RIVM is in week blocks, the number of hospital admissions and the mortality was evenly distributed across the week days. From these calculations it became apparent that "normal" business continuity could not be maintained for public health services in case of admission of excess numbers of patients with ILI. Obviously, it was also apparent that acute care had to continue for all hospitals. Analysis of hospital admission data showed a 30% contribution of acute care patients on capacity of hospital and ICU beds. The bottleneck in caring for patients with ILI will be at the level of ICU capacity. In their study in European ICUs, Miranda et al showed that mean occupancy rate of ICUs was only 70% and the predominant use of ICU beds was post-operative care, e.g. patients from the operating theatre after planned surgery [88,164,165]. We showed that a major opportunity in creating capacity for ILI patients in hospitals is a temporary admission stop for all post-operative care and general medical patients [160]. This admission stop would have to be in place in advance of the first confirmed patients with ILI. Because it is expected an influenza pandemic will reach Europe approximately two weeks after first confirmed human-to-human transmission in South-East-Asia, clearing all hospitals from post-operative and general medical care patients would have to start at this moment, because analysis of hospital admission data showed a maximum length of stay of these patients in all hospitals of twelve days. The effect of intensified treatment decisions at patient level on the peak occupancy rate of ICU beds was incorporated in the model. A 48-hour restriction of treatment time at the ICU for 5 and 20% of the patients occupying an ICU bed was applied in the model. The ethical impact on the clinicians and nurses who have to make these decisions was generally recognized. Many clinicians now realize that end-of-life decisions are an integral part of health care which is independent of any specific religious background or culture [166,167]. Intensive-care physicians in The Netherlands have been trained to take charge of decision processes about forgoing life support in the ICU [166]. They have been familiarized with the difficulties in communicating with members of the

ICU team including medical, nursing and technical staff in decisions at the end of life. The challenge during an outbreak of pandemic influenza will be in orchestrating and implementing these decisions under extreme time pressure. Relatives of patients as well as team members may need more time than available to accept that some patients on life support not responding to treatment will not recover. Some may insist on continuation of support although it would be unwise and disrespectful to these patients to continue futile treatment, and unfair to others whose life might have been saved. A subtle and time-consuming approach may not apply under anticipated extreme conditions of pandemic influenza [166]. Decision rules have to be adapted to real-time information updates, from hospital management, obtained during the course of the pandemic, and briefings and exchange of information throughout the pandemic crisis is pivotal. Existing guidelines and protocols like the Pneumonia Severity Index or its modification recommended by the ATS, or the British CURB-65, propagated by the BTS may not apply fully but can be used initially to guide patient management [168].

Chapter 20

WORKFORCE

The possibility of absenteeism of HCWs either due to illness or to care duties at home or in their individual social environment was also incorporated in the model. It was assumed that HCWs will fall ill at a similar rate as the normal population. Although morale has was high during the SARS outbreak in Singapore and Toronto [40], some examples of strained professional behaviour have been reported [47]. We believe that erosion of professionalism and morale may be partly preventable by implementing effective protection for HCW, with appropriate training to comply with protocols for personal protection [45,169]. Length of stay of individual patients in ICUs is the most predominant factor in capacity planning for a pandemic. We showed that, for a worst case scenario of patients kept in the ICU for 15 days, demand for workload and ICU beds exceeds capacity [156,157]. Reducing the length of stay of individual patients will increase the capability of hospitals to serve most ILI patients. ICU nurses and physicians are key HCWs in caring for ILI patients admitted to an ICU. Research showed ICU workload is made up of only 30% of technical, ICU patient stay, related work [93,95,96,165,170]. The majority of workload comprises hygiene procedures, mobilization, support and care of relatives, and administrative and managerial tasks. Insight in workload of ICU nurses and other HCWs' rigorous task differentiation can be obtained and even specific tasks can be delegated to non-HCWs' specialists (for example, communication with family members of deceased patients can be done by spokespersons and communications experts of the individual hospitals) [157]. In this study the smallest gain in available workforce was gained with 8 weeks pre-prophylactic use of neuraminidase inhibitors. Although prophylactic use of neuraminidase inhibitors serves an import role in staff protection and will most likely enhance compliance of HCWs, it serves its role specifically at individual HCW level and not so much on workload level [171]. The largest gain in increasing the number of HCWs will be by expanding the work shift from 8 to 12 hours; this would increase the number of operational HCWs by ≈50%. This will place a huge strain on personnel which is justified, when one considers the relatively short peak surge period, and we expect HCWs to comply.

Expanding the number of available HCWs is also achieved if all general medical and surgical patients are cleared from all fifteen hospitals in the northern part of the Netherlands, 932 medical specialists (anesthesiologists, surgeons, internal medicine, cardiologists and cardio-thoracic surgeons) can be reallocated to see acute care and influenza patients, greatly enhancing the number of HCWs for public health services. Finally, the UMCG has 2,470 undergraduate and graduate medical students, 367 dentistry students and 423 students' movement sciences in 2006. There are also 1,240 Nursing Sciences students and 2,391 students Health Sciences at the Hanze University Groningen of Applied Sciences. If indeed 44.3% (226 out of 510 medical students) of health care related students will report for duty in case of HCW shortage, 3,053 extra HCWs can be recruited for duty during a pandemic to fill the potential gaps in health care delivery [172]. These students can be distributed among all public health services, including general practitioners, in the region.

In a questionnaire study to *willingness* and *ability* of HCWs to report for duty during pandemic influenza, we found approximately 50% of all HCWs reported they would always report for duty [158]. Indeed, the respondents stated if the hospital would provide support in day care for children, care for children if the became sick, provide training to increase self efficacy and provide precautionary measures to (non-)HCWs to prohibit infecting children or spouses would increase compliance among (non-)HCWs to almost 95%.

Chapter 21

GENERAL PRACTITIONERS

General practitioners will play a key role in controlling disease outbreaks. As can be seen from table 1, the models used in The Netherlands, presume a hospital admission rate of 0.3%. Under this assumption, health care services can provide all required care for non-ILI-acute patients and ILI patients during a disease outbreak. This encompasses general practitioners, who are familiar with their population and individual patients will have to apply strict triage decisions, only admitting patients to health services that they believe will benefit most, leaving patients to be cared for at home or in other care facilities that do not benefit from hospital admission. General practitioners therefore need insight in all available health services capacity at any moment in time during a disease outbreak.

Chapter 22

AGE DISTRIBUTION

The UMCG is the only hospital in the region with pediatric hospital and pediatric ICU beds (PICU). We show that an influenza pandemic for children can be managed; even allowing emergency care for non–ILI-related acute cases, only when firm decision-making rules are followed and antiviral therapy is used [159]. The UMCG has 100 pediatric hospital beds of which 70 could be made available for ILI-related hospital admissions. If the attack rate reaches a maximum of 50% with a mean length of stay of 15 hospital days per child, without any additional change in patient management, this would lead to a peak of 282 occupied regular pediatric hospital beds in the age group below 18 years, which would suffice for regular ILI-related acute care. The bottleneck in caring for children in a single center would be PICU capacity. On the basis of results from a semi structured telephone interview with ICU medical staff in the UMCG, a maximum of 31 (of a total of 46) PICU beds could be dedicated to ILI-related acute-care patients, if all post-operative and planned general medical care admissions for children would be postponed. If all children in the age group below 18 years would be admitted to the PICU, with an estimated attack rate of 30%, and 50% PICU admission rate; and a mean length of stay of 8 days, a shortage of 32 PICU bed at day 28 after onset would follow. PICU capacity is extremely limited in the northern part of The Netherlands. This shortage of PICU capacity is exacerbated with any increase in hospital length of stay or ICU length of stay. If only smaller children were allowed to be admitted to PICU and older children would be admitted to adult ICUs and if the full capacity of all 31 PICU beds can be utilized, a shortage of 1 PICU bed at day 28 after onset would follow. For ICU resources, most adult ICUs would be able to technically manage children of 25 kg and over; smaller children require different equipment and disposables. Adult ICUs are therefore equipped to handle patients weighing 25 kg and over. In the Netherlands boys aged 7 and girls aged 8 are expected to weigh about 25 kilograms and hence can be admitted to an adult ICU.

It is recognized this has a tremendous impact on the pediatric clinicians and nurses who have to make these triage decisions [25,72,108].

Chapter 23

UNDERLYING DISEASE AND CO-MORBIDITY

During a pandemic, individuals with severe co-morbidities may opt for supportive care without hospital and/or ICU admission, in consultation with their loved ones, and their general practitioners. A large proportion of these individuals may very well die because of ILI. This will place an unusual high strain on general practitioners who would have to make triage decisions and who would have to communicate with the relatives.

Chapter 24

MITIGATION AND CONTAINMENT MEASURES FOR PANDEMIC INFLUENZA

In the models the effect of treatment (within 48 hours of infection) with antiviral medication on the spread and the impact of the pandemic was considered [74,86]. Antiviral medication is assumed to reduce the total number of hospital admissions by 50% and mortality by around 30%. In the hospital protocols for management of patients of pandemic influenza and other high-risk respiratory pathogens, extensive measures are included to separate ILI patients from other patients and focus on the protection of staff [79]. Adherence to similar protocols has been shown to protect HCWs caring for patients with SARS [169]. Public health care services protocols in the northern part of The Netherlands comprise of three major rules: protection of HCWs staff, protection of other acute care patients and optimum care for ILI patients including quarantine and isolation protocols.

The effect of antiviral medications, vaccination campaigns and, for instance closure of schools and airports may alter the key characteristics of the pandemic, all having the effect that onset is delayed and that the course is more protracted, with a much lower peak in incident cases [84]. Even a less than perfect vaccine might have a tremendous impact on the course of the pandemic. Stock-piling is now implemented for influenza A/H5N1 to be able to produce vast quantities of vaccine with a limited protection potential against the new virus. In the Netherlands, stock piling of oseltamivir has been implemented, both for the public at large and for health care facilities and HCW working at the front line during the flu pandemic. Stockpiling of antimicrobials to combat secondary bacterial pneumonia is yet another important logistic challenge [173].

Chapter 25

METHODOLOGICAL CONSIDERATIONS

There are limitations to the analyses and model that we developed and used here. The models are based on incomplete and sometimes conflicting or inconsistent information on the impact of an influenza pandemic. It is assumed that more reliable data will only become available when the pandemic is in progress. The need for surge capacity of hospital resources is more dependent on the combination of excess hospital admissions and length of stay than the mere number of hospital admissions. The small percentage of patients admitted to hospital in the models (based on past experiences) implies that relatively small increases in admittance rate will have a huge impact on public health services resources requirement. The report by the Writing Committee of the Second WHO on Clinical Aspects of Human Infection with Avian Influenza [22] prompts us to discuss the impact these findings have on preparedness planning of health care organizations. The case fatality rate of 61% in total, especially among persons aged 10 to 19 years and the much lower rate in persons aged 50 years of age or older is different from what has been learned from past pandemics [30,37,109]. This increased case fatality rate among the age group 10 to 19 years will have a tremendous impact on hospital and health care institutions pandemic preparedness planning and the models presented here. In the prevailing modelling it is assumed that persons between 10 and 19 years only make up a small percentage of potential hospitalized persons [156]. The question that has not been answered by the Writing Committee is whether this age group is at particular risk or whether this is because this age group is mainly responsible for handling poultry and poultry products in reports on avian influenza. In the Netherlands, there are approximately two million persons between the age of 10 and 19 years on a total of 16.4 million inhabitants (12%). The same proportion holds for the 27 countries of the European Union (494 million inhabitants, 57 million persons between 10 and 19 years of age, 11.7%).

In affluent countries preparation for a pandemic is mostly supported and financed at national level and the overall assumption is that health care services capacity will suffice. Less affluent countries might have more difficulties with pandemic preparation. For affluent countries, the economic ramifications of "loosing" the younger generation struck by avian influenza might be even more dramatic then a pandemic it self because affluent countries are dealing with an increasing older population and affluent countries, with lower birth rates, value children tremendously. Loss of children would be a terrible blow to morale and would influence resilience. The models used for calculating workload demand are based on the datasets of the EURICUS-projects and were these studies date back almost a decade ago. Because of changes in ICU technology and professional changes within ICU nursing practice, with decreasing emphasis on technical procedures, and increased emphasis on communication within the ICU team and communication with the patients' relatives, some variables like NEMS [95] (change in workload), Length of Stay (LOS) and ICU mortality may have changed. We expect that the models present a worst-case scenario for ICU admissions and workload.

Chapter 26

CONCLUSION

Modelling impact of disease outbreaks and EBM needs to be followed by EBMgt of health care services. This includes using disease outbreaks models and knowledge about surge capacity on regional, national and international level, to ensure business continuity. Business continuity also encompasses ethical decisions (use of surge capacity) and finances. EBM and EBMgt decision rules have to be adapted to real-time information updates obtained during the course of a disease outbreak and exchange of information throughout the crisis is pivotal. Sharing of company sensitive information (e.g. number of available hospital and ICU beds, occupancy rate, and number of HCWs) and recognition of mutual dependency has resulted in the development of a "capacity monitor", an on-line real-time internet database containing all necessary available data, which can be consulted by all management and HCWs involved in patient care during pandemic influenza. Using EBMgt, *mindful* (e.g. of the effectiveness or ineffectiveness of the methods to be chosen to achieve an objective); and *critical* (e.g. of the underlying assumptions of the methods); *profoundly simple* and *common sense* decisions can be made by the management of public health services to provide the context for key HCWs to focus on the content of caring for ILI patients. Models should be used as an integral part of preparedness plans.

Overall assessment that a influenza pandemic with assumptions described here, can be managed and controlled at the level of health care institutions clearly contrasts with the sobering and daunting analysis presented for ICU capacity in the United Kingdom or Australasia [86,97]. In the models presented in this chapter it is shown that business continuity is maintainable when strict, clear and disciplined hierarchical structures are in place.

Based on the findings the following recommendations can be made:

Recommendation one: Implement EBMgt for public health service managers. Only management can prepare the context in which care for ILI patients has to be delivered. This also involves facing the hard facts and dealing with inconsistent and sometimes conflicting information.;

Recommendation two: Start preparations in time, when WHO declares Phase IV, stop all post-operative care and general medical admissions. Clear hospital beds and free HCWs. If hospitals are not cleared there will not only be not enough hospital and ICU beds available for ILI patients, also unnecessary risk of exposure to ILI will be placed on these patients.;

Recommendation three: Implement a simple nursing workload measurement system for scarce resources. This will provide valuable information on the current workload and will aid in planning for a pandemic. [92,133,164,174];

Recommendation four: Gain insight, per health care service, in general and acute care population. This will give insight in the number of hospital and ICU beds and the number of HCWs capable of being cleared for ILI patients.

Recommendation five: Children between the ages of 7 and 18 years should be admitted to adult ICUs as PICU capacity will be insufficient.; therefore;

Recommendation six: PICU Physicians and Nurses should be prepared and trained to assist for care to be delivered in adult surgical, medical and mixed ICUs, and familiarize with the adult ICU setting and environment.;

Recommendation seven: Strict and clear triage decisions must be in place, with clear decision rules combined with clinical expertise so as to distribute fair chances for the majority of ILI-afflicted children.;

Recommendation eight: Rigorous task differentiation, clear hierarchical management, unambiguous communication and discipline are essential and we recommend informing and training non-ICU HCWs for possible duties at the ICU. Their training should address the needs of ICU HCWs, and family and loved ones of individuals admitted to the ICU with ILI. It should also incorporate the potential difficulties in communication of HCWs with family members and loved ones if patients die after intensified treatment decisions .[156,175,176];

Recommendation nine: Sharing of business sensitive information between all public health services and the notion of mutually dependency and fair share of the strain of caring for the population is essential and should be implemented before a disease outbreak is an actuality.

ACKNOWLEDGEMENT

We thank Prof. dr. A. (Addie) Johnson PhD, Professor of Work and Experimental Psychology at the University of Groningen, the Netherlands, for critical review of the manuscript and providing us with helpful comments.

REFERENCES

[1] Abdel-Ghafar, A.N., Chotpitayasunondh, T., Gao, Z., Hayden, F.G., Nguyen, D.H., de Jong, M.D., Naghdaliyev, A., Peiris, J.S., Shindo, N., Soeroso, S. & Uyeki, T.M. (2008). Update on avian influenza A (H5N1) virus infection in humans. *N. Engl. J. Med. 358*, 261-273

[2] Abikusno, N. (2006). Bird flu in Indonesia. *Bird flu: a rising pandemic in Asia and beyond? 1*, 85-97

[3] Anonymous. (2005). Evolution of H5N1 avian influenza viruses in Asia. *Emerg. Infec.t Dis. 11*, 1515-1521

[4] Beigel, J.H., Farrar, J. & Han, A.M. (2005). (The Writing Committee of the World Health Organisation (WHO) Consultation on Human Influenza A/H5). Avian influenza A(H5N1) infection in humans. *N. Eng. J. Med. 353*, 373-385

[5] Boender, G., Hagenaars,T., Bouma, A., Nodelijk, G., Elbers, A., de Jong, M. & van Boven, M. (2007). Risk Maps for the Spread of Highly Pathogenic Avian Influenza in Poultry. *PLoS Comput. Biol. 3*, e71

[6] Chai, L.Y. A. (2006). Avian influenza: basic science, potential for mutation, transmission, illness symptomatology and vaccines. *Bird flu: a rising pandemic in Asia and beyond? 1*, 1-13

[7] Chan, P.K. (2002). Outbreak of avian influenza A(H5N1) virus infection in Hong Kong in 1997. *Clin. Infect. Dis. 34 Suppl 2*, S58-S64

[8] Claas, E.C., Osterhaus, A.D., van Beek, R., de Jong, J.C., Rimmelzwaan, G.F., Senne, D.A. & et al. (1998). Human influenza A H5N1 virus related to a highly pathogenic avian influenza virus. *Lancet. 351*, 472-477

[9] Colizza, V., Barrat, A., Barthelemy, M., Valleron, A.J. & Vespignani, A. (2007). Modeling the Worldwide Spread of Pandemic Influenza: Baseline Case and Containment Interventions. *PLoS Medicine. 4*, e13

[10] de Jong, M.D., Simmons, C.P., Thanh, T.T., Hien, V.M., Smith, G.J.D., Chau, T.N.B., Hoang, D.M., Vinh Chau, N., Khanh, T.H., Dong, V.C., Qui, P.T., Van Cam, B., Ha, D. Q., Guan, Y., Peiris, J.S.M., Chinh, N.T., Hien, T.T. & Farrar, J. (2006). Fatal outcome of human influenza A (H5N1) is associated with high viral load and hypercytokinemia. *Nat. Med. 12*, 1203-1207

[11] Ferguson, N. M., Cummings, D.A.T. & Cauchemez, S. (2005). Strategies for containing an emerging influenza pandemic in Southeast Asia. *Nature. 437*, 209-214

[12] Kandun, I.N., Wibisono, H., Sedyaningsih, E.R., Yusharmen, Hadisoedarsuno, W., Purba, W., Santoso, H., Septiawati, C., Tresnaningsih, E., Heriyanto, B., Yuwono, D., Harun, S., Soeroso, S., Giriputra, S., Blair, P.J., Jeremijenko, A., Kosasih, H., Putnam, S.D., Samaan, G., Silitonga, M., Chan, K.H., Poon, L.L.M., Lim, W., Klimov, A., Lindstrom, S., Guan, Y., Donis, R., Katz, J., Cox, N., Peiris, M. & Uyeki, T.M. (2006). Three Indonesian Clusters of H5N1 Virus Infection in 2005. *N. Engl. J. Med. 355*, 2186-2194

[13] Kilpatrick, A.M., Chmura, A.A., Gibbons, D.W., Fleischer, R.C., Marra, P.P. & Daszak, P. (2006). From the Cover: Predicting the global spread of H5N1 avian influenza. *Proc. Natl. Acad. Sci. U.S.A. 103*, 19368-19373

[14] Koh, G.C.H., Wong, T.Y., Cheong, S.K. & Koh, D.S.Q. (2008). Avian Influenza: a global threat needing a global solution. *Asia Pac. Fam. Med. 7*, 5

[15] Schunemann, H.J., Hill, S.R. & Kakad, M. (2007). WHO Rapid Advice Guidelines for pharmacological management of sporadic human infection with avian influenza (H5N1) virus. *Lancet Infect. Dis. 7*, 21-31

[16] Stohr, K. (2005). Avian influenza and pandemics - research needs and opportunities. *N. Engl. J. Med. 352*, 405-407

[17] The Writing Committee of the World Health Organization (WHO) Consultation on Human Influenza. (2005). Avian Influenza A (H5N1) Infection in Humans. *N. Engl. J. Med. 353*, 1374-1385

[18] Tracy, C. S., Upshur, R.E. & Daar, A.S. (2005). Avian influenza and pandemics. *N. Engl. J. Med. 352*, 1928

[19] Webster, R. & Govorkova, E. (2006). H5N1 Influenza -- Continuing Evolution and Spread. *N. Engl. J. Med. 355*, 2174-2177

[20] Winker, K., McCracken, K.G., Gibson, D.D., Pruett, C.L., Meier, R. & Huettmann, F. (2007). Movements of birds and avian influenza from Asia into Alaska. *Emerg. Infect. Dis. 13*, 547-552
[21] World Health Organization. (2008). Cumulative Number of Confirmed Human Cases of Avian Influenza A/(H5N1) Reported to WHO. *http://www who int/csr/disease/avian_influenza/country/ cases_table_ 2008_06_19/en/index html.*
[22] Writing Committee of the Second World Health Organization Consultation on Clinical Aspects of Human Infection with Avian Influenza. (2008). Update on Avian Influenza A (H5N1) Virus Infection in Humans. *N. Engl. J. Med. 358*, 261-273
[23] Taubenberger, J. K. & Morens, D.M. (2006). 1918 Influenza: the Mother of All Pandemics. *Emerg. Infect. Dis. 12*, 15-22
[24] Ahmed, R., Oldstone, M.B.A. & Palese, P. (2007). Protective immunity and susceptibility to infectious diseases: lessons from the 1918 influenza pandemic. *Nat. Immunol. 8*, 1188-1193
[25] Brundage, J.F. & Shanks G.D. (2008). Deaths from bacterial pneumonia during 1918–19 influenza pandemic. *Emerg. Infect. Dis. 14*, 1193-1199
[26] Brundage, J. F. (2006). Cases and deaths during influenza pandemics in the United States. *Am. J. Prev. Med. 31*, 252-256
[27] Kash, J., Tumpey,T., Proll,S., Carter,V., Perwitasari,O., Thomas,M., Basler,C., Palese,P., Taubenberger,J., Garcia-Sastre,A., Swayne,D. & Katze,M. (2006). Genomic analysis of increased host immune and cell death responses induced by 1918 influenza virus. *Nature. 443*, 578-581
[28] Kilbourne, E. D. (2006). Influenza pandemics of the 20th century. *Emerg. Infect. Dis. 12*, 9-14
[29] Kobasa, D., Jones, S., Shinya, K., Kash, J., Copps, J., Ebihara, H., Hatta, Y., Hyun Kim,J., Halfmann,P., Hatta,M., Feldmann,F., Alimonti,J., Fernando,L., Li,Y., Katze,M., Feldmann,H. & Kawaoka,Y. (2007). Aberrant innate immune response in lethal infection of macaques with the 1918 influenza virus. *Nature. 445*, 319-323
[30] Langford, C. (2002). The Age Pattern of Mortality in the 1918-19 Influenza Pandemic: An Attempted Explanation Based on Data for England and Wales. *Med. Hist. 46*, 1-20
[31] Palese, P., Tumpey,T.M. & Garcia-Sastre,A. (2006). What Can We Learn from Reconstructing the Extinct 1918 Pandemic Influenza Virus? *Immunity. 24*, 121-124

[32] Reid, A. H., Fanning,T.G., Janczewski,T.A. & Taubenberger,J.K. (2000). Characterization of the 1918 "Spanish" influenza virus neuraminidase gene. *Proc. Natl. Acad. Sci. U.S.A. 97*, 6785-6790

[33] Tumpey, T., Basler,C., Aguilar,P., Zeng,H., Solorzano,A., Swayne,D., Cox,N., Katz,J., Taubenberger,J., Palese,P. & Garcia-Sastre,A. (2005). Characterization of the Reconstructed 1918 Spanish Influenza Pandemic Virus. *Science. 310*, 77-80

[34] Chowell, G., Ammon,C.E., Hengartner,N.W. & Hyman,J.M. (2006). Transmission dynamics of the great influenza pandemic of 1918 in Geneva, Switzerland: Assessing the effects of hypothetical interventions. *J. Theor. Biol. 241*, 193-204

[35] Hatchett, R., Mecher,C. & Lipsitch,M. (2007). From the Cover: Public health interventions and epidemic intensity during the 1918 influenza pandemic. *Proc. Natl. Acad. Sci. U.S.A. 104*, 7582-7587

[36] Hart, J.C. (2008). The 1957 Asian influenza epidemic. 1958. *Conn. Med. 72*, 107-113

[37] Viboud, C., Tam,T., Fleming,D., Handel,A., Miller,M. & Simonsen,L. (2006). Transmissibility and mortality impact of epidemic and pandemic influenza, with emphasis on the unusually deadly 1951 epidemic. *Vaccine. 24*, 6701-6707

[38] Sprenger, M.J., Mulder, P.G., Beyer, W.E., van Strik, R. & Masurel, N. (1993). Impact of influenza on mortality in relation to age and underlying disease, 1967-1989. *Int. J. Epidemiol. 22*, 334-340

[39] Anderson, R. M., Fraser, C. & Ghani, A.C. (2004). Epidemiology, transmission dynamics and control of SARS: the 2002-2003 epidemic. *Philos Trans. R Soc. Lond. B Biol. Sci. 359*, 1091-1105

[40] Bournes, D.A. & Ferguson-Pare, M. (2005). Persevering Through a Difficult Time During the SARS Outbreak in Toronto. *Nurs. Sci. Q. 18*, 324-333

[41] Emanuel, E. J. (2003). The lessons of SARS. *Ann. Intern. Med. 139*, 589-591

[42] Finlay, B., See, R. & Brunham, R. (2004). Rapid response research to emerging infectious diseases: lessons from SARS. *Nat. Rev. Micro. 2*, 602-607

[43] Gommans, J. (2003). Coping with severe acute respiratory syndrome: a personal view of the good, the bad and the ugly. *N. Z. Med. J. 116*, U465

[44] Hsin, D. H. & Macer, D.R. (2004). Heroes of SARS: professional roles and ethics of health care workers. *J. Infect. 49*, 210-215

References

[45] Loeb, M., McGeer, A., Henry, B., Ofner, M., Rose, D., Hlywka, T. & et al. (2004). SARS among critical care nurses, Toronto. *Emerg. Infect. Dis. 10*, 251-255

[46] Singer, P.A., Benatar, S.R., Bernstein, M., Daar, A.S., Dickens, B.M., MacRae,S.K., Upshur,R.E., Wright,L. & Shaul,R.Z. (2003). Ethics and SARS: lessons from Toronto. *BMJ. 327*, 1342-1344

[47] Straus, S.E., Wilson, K., Rambaldini, G., Rath, D., Lin, Y., Gold, W.L. & Kapral, M.K. (2004). Severe acute respiratory syndrome and its impact on professionalism: qualitative study of physicians' behaviour during an emerging healthcare crisis. *BMJ. 329*, 83

[48] Wenzel, R. P. & Edmond, M.B. (2003). Managing SARS amidst uncertainty. *N. Engl. J. Med. 348*, 1947-1948

[49] World Health Organization. Summary of probable SARS cases with onset of illness from 1 November 2002 to 31 July 2003. 2007. [cited 2009 April 12]. Available from: *http://www.who.int/csr/sars/country /table2004_04_21/en/index.html*.

[50] Reid, L. (2005). Diminishing returns? Risk and the duty to care in the SARS epidemic. *Bioethics. 19*, 348-361

[51] Matrosovich, M.N., Matrosovich,T.Y., Gray,T., Roberts,N.A. & Klenk,H.D. (2004). Human and avian influenza viruses target different cell types in cultures of human airway epithelium. *Proc. Natl. Acad. Sci. USA. 101*, 4620-4624

[52] van Riel, D., Munster,V.J., de Wit,E., Rimmelzwaan,G.F., Fouchier,R.A.M., Osterhaus,A.D.M.E. & Kuiken,T. (2006). H5N1 Virus Attachment to Lower Respiratory Tract. *Science. 312*, 399

[53] de Jong, M.D., Cam, BV, Qui, P.T., Hien, V.M., Thanh, T.T., Hue, N.B., Beld, M., Phuong, L.T., Khanh, T.H., Chau, N.V.V., Hien, T.T., Ha, D.Q. & Farrar, J. (2005). Fatal Avian Influenza A (H5N1) in a Child Presenting with Diarrhea Followed by Coma. *N. Engl. J. Med. 352*, 686-691

[54] Gabriel, G., Dauber, B., Wolff, T., Planz, O., Klenk, H.D. & Stech, J. (2005). The viral polymerase mediates adaptation of an avian influenza virus to a mammalian host. *Proc. Natl. Acad. Sci. U.S.A. 102*, 18590-18595

[55] Maines, T. R., Chen,L.M., Matsuoka,Y., Chen,H., Rowe,T., Ortin,J., Falcon,A., Hien,N.T., Mai,L.Q., Sedyaningsih,E.R., Harun,S., Tumpey,T.M., Donis,R.O., Cox,N.J., Subbarao,K. & Katz,J.M. (2006). Lack of transmission of H5N1 avian-human reassortant influenza viruses in a ferret model. *Proc. Natl. Acad. Sci. U.S.A. 103*, 12121-12126

[56] Gill, J.S., Webby, R., Gilchrist, M.J. & Gray, G.C. (2006). Avian influenza among waterfowl hunters and wildlife professionals. *Emerg. Infect. Dis. 12*, 1284-1286
[57] Ci-yong, L., Jia-hai, L., Wei-qing, C., Li-fang, J., Bing-yan, T., Wen-hua, L., Bo-jian, Z. & Hong-yan, S. (2008). Potential infections of H5N1 and H9N2 avian influenza do exist in Guangdong populations of China. *Chin. Med. J. 121*, 2050-2053
[58] Katz, J.M., Lim, W., Bridges, C.B., Rowe, T., Hu-Primmer, J., Lu, X. & et al. (1999). Antibody response in individuals infected with avian influenza A (H5N1) viruses and detection of anti-H5 antibody among household and social contacts. *J. Infect. Dis. 180*, 1763-1770
[59] Meijer, A., Bosman, A., van de Kamp, E.E., Wilbrink, B., du Ry van Beest Holle, M. & Koopmans, M. (2006). Measurement of antibodies to avian influenza virus A (H7N7) in humans by hemagglutination inhibition test. *J. Virol. Methods. 132*, 113-120
[60] Terregino, C., Cattoli,G., De Nardi,R., Beato,M.S., Capua,I., Guberti,V. & Scremin,M. (2005). Isolation of influenza A viruses subtype H7N7 and H7N4 from waterfowl in Italy. *Vet. Rec. 156*, 292-29a
[61] Fouchier, R.A., Schneeberger, P.M., Rozendaal, F.W., Broekman, J.M., Kemink, S.A., Munster, V. & et al. (2004). Avian influenza A virus (H7N7) associated with human conjunctivitis and a fatal case of acute respiratory distress syndrome. *Proc. Natl. Acad. Sci. U.S.A. 101*, 1356-1361
[62] Koopmans, M., Wilbrink B., Conyn M., Natrop G., van der Nat H., Vennema H. & et al. (2004). Transmission of H7N7 avian influenza A virus to human beings during a large outbreak in commercial poultry farms in the Netherlands. *Lancet. 363*, 587-593
[63] Peiris, J.S., Yu, W.C., Leung, C.W., Cheung, C.Y., Ng, W.F., Nicholls, J.M. & et al. (2004). Re-emergence of fatal human influenza A subtype H5N1 disease. *Lancet. 363*, 617-619
[64] European Commission Health & Consumer Protection Directorate General. A report on surveys for avian influenza in poultry in member states during 2005. 2005 [cited 2009 April 12]. Available from: *http://ec.europa.eu/food/animal/diseases/controlmeasures/avian/res_ai_ surv_poultry_2005_en pdf.*
[65] Keawcharoen, J., van Riel,D., van Amerongen,G., Bestebroer,T., Beyer,W.E. & van Lavieren,R. (2008). Wild ducks as long-distance vectors of highly pathogenic avian influenza virus (H5N1). *Emerg. Infect. Dis. 14*, 600-607

[66] Olsen, B., Munster,V.J., Wallensten,A., Waldenstrom,J., Osterhaus,A.D. & Fouchier,R.A. (2006). Global patterns of influenza a virus in wild birds. *Science. 312*, 384-388
[67] Anonymous. (1998). Randomised trial of efficacy and safety of inhaled zanamivir in treatment of influenza A and B virus infections. The MIST (Management of Influenza in the Southern Hemisphere Trialists) Study Group. *Lancet. 352*, 1877-1881
[68] Normille, D. & Enserink, M. (2007). Avian influenza: with change in the seasons, bird flu returns. *Science. 315*, 448
[69] Reid, A. H., Fanning,T.G., Hultin,J.V. & Taubenberger,J.K. (1999). Origin and evolution of the 1918 "Spanish" influenza virus hemagglutinin gene. *Proc. Natl. Acad. Sci. U.S.A. 96*, 1651-1656
[70] Reid, A. H., Fanning,T.G., Janczewski,T.A., McCall,S. & Taubenberger,J.K. (2002). Characterization of the 1918 "Spanish" influenza virus matrix gene segment. *J. Virol. 76*, 10717-10723
[71] Reid, A. H., Fanning,T.G., Janczewski,T.A., Lourens,R.M. & Taubenberger,J.K. (2004). Novel origin of the 1918 pandemic influenza virus nucleoprotein gene. *J. Virol. 78*, 12462-12470
[72] Gupta, R.K., George, R. & Nguyen-Van-Tam, J.S. (2008). Bacterial pneumonia and pandemic influenza planning. *Emerg. Infect. Dis. 14*, 1187-1192
[73] Morens, D. M., Taubenberger, J.K. & Fauci,A.S. (2008). Predominant Role of Bacterial Pneumonia as a Cause of Death in Pandemic Influenza: Implications for Pandemic Influenza Preparedness. *J. Infect. Dis. 198*, 962-970
[74] Nordstrom, B.L., Sung, I., Suter, P. & Szneke, P. (2005). Risk of pneumonia and other complications of influenza-like illness in patients treated with oseltamivir. *Curr. Med. Res. Opin. 21*, 761-768
[75] Smitherman, H. F., Caviness, A.C. & Macias,C.G. (2005). Retrospective Review of Serious Bacterial Infections in Infants Who Are 0 to 36 Months of Age and Have Influenza A Infection. *Pediatrics. 115*, 710-718
[76] Krauss, H., Weber A., Appel M., Enders B., v.Graevenitz A., Isenberg H.D., Schiefer H.G., Slenczka W. & Zahner H. (2003). *Zoonoses. Infectious Diseases Transmissible from Animals to Humans.* (3rd). Washington DC, USA: ASM Press. American Society for Microbiology.
[77] Cinti, S. (2005). Pandemic Influenza: Are We Ready? *Disaster Management & Response. 3*, 61-67

[78] Van Genugten, M.L.L., Heijnen M.L.A. & Jager J.C. (2003). Pandemic Influenza and Healthcare Demand in the Netherlands: Scenario Analysis. *Emerg. Infect. Dis. 9*, 531-538
[79] Bartlett, J.G. (2006). Planning for avian influenza. *Ann. Intern. Med. 145*, 141-144
[80] Beigel, J.H., Farrar, J., Han, A.M., Hayden, F.G., Hyer, R., de Jong, M.D. & et al. (2005). Avian influenza A (H5N1) infection in humans. *N Engl. J. Med. 353*, 1374-1385
[81] Fauci, A.S. (2006). Pandemic influenza threat and preparedness. *Emerg Infect Dis. 12*, 73-77
[82] Tsang, K.W., Eng, P., Liam, C.K., Shim, Y.S. & Lam, W.K. (2005). H5N1 influenza pandemic: contingency plans. *Lancet. 366*, 533-534
[83] Nicoll, A. (2006). Human H5N1 infections: so many cases - why so little knowledge? *Euro Surveill. 11*,
[84] Ferguson, N.M., Cummings, D.A.T., Fraser, C., Cajka, J.C., Cooley, P.C. & Burke, D.S. (2006). Strategies for mitigating an influenza pandemic. *Nature. 442*, 448-452
[85] Gruber, P.C., Gomersall, C.D. & Joynt, G.M. (2006). Avian influenza (H5N1): implications for intensive care. *Intens Care Med. 32*, 823-829
[86] Menon, D.K., Taylor, B.L. & Ridley, S.A. (2005). Modelling the impact of an influenza pandemic on critical care services in England. *Anaesthesia. 60*, 952-954
[87] Hagenaars, T.J., Van Genugten, M.L.L. & Wallinga, J. (2003). Scenario analysis of transmission dynamics, health-care demand and mortality. *Brief report to the Health Inspectorate of the Netherlands*,
[88] Miranda, D.R., Ryan, D., Schaufeli, W.B. & Fidler, V. (1997). *Organisation and Management of Intensive Care: A prospective study in 12 European Countries*. Berlin: Springer Verlag.
[89] Iapichino, G., Radrizzani, D., Bertolini, G., Ferla, L., Pasetti, G., Pezzi, A., Porta, F. & Miranda, D.R. (2001). Daily classification of the level of care. A method to describe clinical course of illness, use of resources and quality of intensive care assistance. *Intens. Care Med. 27*, 131-136
[90] Iapichino, G., Gattiononi, L., Radrizzani, D., Simini, B., Bertolini,G., Ferla, L., Mostraletti, G., Porta, F. & Miranda, D.R. (2003). Volume of activity and occupancy-rate in intensive care unit (ICU). Association with mortality. *Intens. Care Med. 29*, S95-S95
[91] Iapichino, G., Morabito, A., Mistraletti, G., Ferla,L., Radrizzani, D. & Miranda, D.R. (2003). Determinants of post-intensive care mortality in high-level treated critically ill patients. *Intens. Care Med. 29*, 1751-1756

[92] Iapichino, G., Mistraletti, G., Corbella, D., Bassi, G., Borotto, E., Miranda, D.R. & Morabito, A. (2006). Scoring system for the selection of high-risk patients in the intensive care unit. *Crit. Care Med. 34*, 1039-1043

[93] Moreno, R., Miranda, D.R., Matos, R. & Fevereiro, T. (2001). Mortality after discharge from intensive care: the impact of organ system failure and nursing workload use at discharge. *Intens. Care Med. 27*, 999-1004

[94] Miranda, D.R., de Rijk, A. & Schaufeli, W. (1996). Simplified Therapeutic Intervention Scoring System: The TISS-28 items - Results from a multicenter study. *Crit. Care Med. 24*, 64-73

[95] Miranda, D.R., Moreno, R. & Iapichino, G. (1997). Nine equivalents of nursing manpower use score (NEMS). *Intens. Care Med. 23*, 760-765

[96] Moreno, R. & Miranda, D.R. (1998). Nursing staff in intensive care in Europe - The mismatch between planning and practice. *Chest. 113*, 752-758

[97] Anderson, T.A., Hart, G.K. & Kainer, M.A. (2003). Pandemic influenza-implications for critical care resources in Australia and New Zealand. *J. Crit. Care. 18*, 173-180

[98] Anantham, D., McHugh, W., O'Neill, S. & Forrow, L. (2008). Clinical review: Influenza pandemic - physicians and their obligations. *Crit. Care. 12*, 217

[99] Bevan, J.C. & Upshur, R.E. (2003). Anesthesia, ethics, and severe acute respiratory syndrome. *Can. J. Anaesth. 50*, 977-979

[100] Ruderman, C., Tracy, C.S., Bensimon, C., Bernstein, M., Hawryluck, L., Shaul, R. & Upshur, R. (2006). On pandemics and the duty to care: whose duty? who cares? *BMC Medical Ethics. 7*, 5

[101] Ehrenstein, B.P. (2008). Pandemic influenza: are we prepared to face our obligations? *Crit. Care. 12*, 165

[102] Ehrenstein, B. P., Hanses, F. & Salzberger, B. (2006). Influenza pandemic and professional duty: family or patients first? A survey of hospital employees. *BMC Public Health. 6*, 311

[103] Qureshi, K., Gershon, R., Sherman, M., Straub, T., Gebbie, E., McCollum, M., Erwin, M. & Morse, S. (2005). Health care workers ability and willingness to report to duty during catastrophic disasters. *Journal of Urban Health. 82*, 378-388

[104] Imai, T., Takahashi, K., Todoroki, M., Kunishima, H., Hoshuyama, T., Ide, R., Kawasaki, T., Koyama, N., Endo, K., Fujita, H., Iwata, K., Koh, G., Chia, S. & Koh, D. (2008). Perception in Relation to a Potential

Influenza Pandemic among Healthcare Workers in Japan: Implications for Preparedness. *J. Occup. Health. 50*, 13-23

[105] Balicer, R. D., Omer, S.B., Barnett, D.J. & Everly, G.S. (2006). Local public health workers' perceptions toward responding to an influenza pandemic. *BMC Public Health. 6*, 99

[106] Masterson, L., Steffen, C., Brin M., Kordick, M.F. & Christos, S. (2009). Willingness to Respond: Of Emergency Department Personnel and Their Predicted Participation in Mass Casualty Terrorist Events. *J. Emerg. Med. 36*, 43-49

[107] Alexander, G. C. & Wynia, M.K. (2003). Ready and willing? Physicians' sense of preparedness for bioterrorism. *Health Aff. (Millwood). 22*, 189-197

[108] Woods, C. R. & Abramson, J.S. (2005). The Next Influenza Pandemic: Will we be Ready to Care for Our Children? *J. Pediatr. 147*, 147-155

[109] Armstrong, G. L., Conn, L.A. & Pinner, R.W. (1999). Trends in Infectious Disease Mortality in the United States During the 20th Century. *JAMA. 281*, 61-66

[110] Miranda, D.R. & Nap, R.E. (2006). The age of the elderly. *Neth. J. Crit. Care. 10*, 621-624

[111] Baltussen, R.M., Reinders, A., Sprenger, M.J.W., Postma, M.J., Jager, J.C., Ament, A.J.H.A. & Leidl, R.M. (1998). Estimating influenza-related hospitalization in the Netherlands. *Epidemiol. Infect. 121*, 129-138

[112] Ilyinskii, P.O., Thoidis, G. & Shneider, A.M. (2008). Development of a vaccine against pandemic influenza viruses: current status and perspectives. *Int. Rev. Immunol. 27*, 392-426

[113] Longini, I. M., Nizam, A. & Xu, S. (2005). Containing pandemic influenza at the source. *Science. 309*, 1083-1087

[114] Osterholm, M. T. (2005). Preparing for the Next Pandemic. *N. Eng. J. Med. 352*, 1839-1842

[115] World Health Organization Writing Group. (2006). Nonpharmaceutical Interventions for Pandemic Influenza, National and Community Measures. *Emerg. Infect. Dis. 12*,

[116] Longini, I., Halloran, M.E., Nizam, A. & Yang, Y. (2004). Containing Pandemic Influenza with Antiviral Agents. *Am. J. Epidemiol. 159*, 623-633

[117] Besselaar, T.G., Naidoo, D., Buys, A., Gregory, V., McAnerney, J., Manamela, J.M. & et al. (2008). Widespread oseltamivir resistance in

influenza A viruses (H1N1), South Africa [letter]. *Emerg. Infect. Dis. 14*, 1809

[118] Kaiser, L., Wat, C., Mills, T., Mahoney, P., Ward, P. & Hayden, F. (2003). Impact of Oseltamivir Treatment on Influenza-Related Lower Respiratory Tract Complications and Hospitalizations. *Arch. Intern. Med. 163*, 1667-1672

[119] Whitley, R. J., Hayden, F.G., Reisinger, K.S., Young, N., Dutkowski, R., Ipe, D., Mills, R.G. & Ward, P. (2001). Oral oseltamivir treatment of influenza in children. *Pediatr. Infect. Dis. J. 20*, 127-133

[120] Ginsberg, J., Mohebbi, M., Patel, R., Brammer, L., Smolinski, M. & Brilliant, L. (2009). Detecting influenza epidemics using search engine query data. *Nature. 457*, 1012-1014

[121] Morse, S. S., Garwin, R.L. & Olsiewski,P.J. (2006). Next flu pandemic: what to do until the vaccine arrives? *Science. 314*, 929

[122] Baras, B., Stittelaar, K.J., Simon, J.H., Thoolen, R.J.M.M., Mossman, S.P., Pistoor, F.H.M., van Amerongen, G., Wettendorff, M.A., Hanon, E. & Osterhaus, A.D.M.E. (2008). Cross-Protection against Lethal H5N1 Challenge in Ferrets with an Adjuvanted Pandemic Influenza Vaccine. *PLoS ONE. 3,*

[123] Carter, N.J. & Plosker, G.L. (2008). Prepandemic influenza vaccine H5N1 (split virion, inactivated, adjuvanted) [Prepandrix]: a review of its use as an active immunization against influenza A subtype H5N1 virus. *BioDrugs. 22*, 279-292

[124] El Sahly, H. & Keitel,W. (2008). Pandemic H5N1 influenza vaccine development: an update. *Expert Rev. Vaccines. 7*, 241-247

[125] Cox, M. & Hollister, J. FluBlok, a next generation influenza vaccine manufactured in insect cells. *Biologicals. In Press, Corrected Proof,*

[126] Sencer, D. J. & Millar,J.D. (2006). Reflections on the 1976 swine flu vaccination program. *Emerg. Infect. Dis. 12*, 29-33

[127] Yamada, T., Dautry, A. & Walport, M. (2008). Ready for avian flu? *Nature. 454*, 162

[128] Leroux-Roels, I., Borkowski, A., Vanwolleghem,T., Drame,M., Clement,F., Hons,E., Devaster,J.M. & Leroux-Roels,G. (2007). Antigen sparing and cross-reactive immunity with an adjuvanted rH5N1 prototype pandemic influenza vaccine: a randomised controlled trial. *Lancet. 370*, 580-589

[129] Stephenson, I., Bugarini,R., Nicholson,K.G., Podda,A., Wood,J.M., Zambon,M.C. & Katz, J.M. (2005). Cross-reactivity to highly pathogenic avian influenza H5N1 viruses after vaccination with

nonadjuvanted and MF59-adjuvanted influenza A/Duck/Singapore/97 (H5N3) vaccine: a potential priming strategy. *J. Infect. Dis. 191*, 1210-1215

[130] Koh, G. C. H. & Koh, D.S.Q. (2006). The socioeconomic effects of an avian influenza pandemic. In Tambyah, P. and Leung, P.C. (Eds.), *Bird flu: a rising pandemic in Asia and beyond?* (1, pp. 127-146). Singapore: World Scientific Publishing.

[131] Smith, K. J. & Roberts, M.S. (2002). Cost-effectiveness of newer treatment strategies for influenza. *Am. J. Med. 113*, 300-307

[132] Barnes, J.C. (2001). *A Guide to Business Continuity Planning*. Chichester: John Wiley & Sons Ltd.

[133] Hick, J.L. & O'Laughlin, D.T. (2006). Concept of Operations for Triage of Mechanical Ventilation in an Epidemic. *Acad. Emerg. Med. 13*, 223-229

[134] Burnet, F. & Clark, E. (1942). Influenza: a survey of the last 50 years in the light of modern work on the virus of epidemic influenza. Melbourne

[135] Frost, W.H. (1920). Statistics of influenza morbidity. *Public Health Rep. 35*, 584-597

[136] Svoboda, T., Henry, B., Shulman, L., Kennedy, E., Rea, E., Ng, W., Wallington, T., Yaffe, B., Gournis, E., Vicencio, E., Basrur, S. & Glazier, R.H. (2004). Public health measures to control the spread of the severe acute respiratory syndrome during the outbreak in Toronto. *N Eng. J. Med. 350*, 2352-2361

[137] Loutfy, M.R., Wallington T., Rutledge T., Mederski B., Rose K., Kwolek S., McRitchie D., Ali A., Wolff B., White D., Glassman E., Ofner M., Low D.E., Berger L., McGeer A., Wong T., Baron D. & Berall G. (2004). Hospital preparedness and SARS. *Emerg. Infect. Dis. 10*, 771-776

[138] Lipshitz, R. (1994). Decision making in three modes. *J. Theor. Soc. Behav. 24*, 47-66

[139] Lipshitz, R. (2007). Paradigms and Mindfulness in Decision Making: Why the Israel Defense Force (I.D.F.) failed in the Second Lebanon War. *Internal Report*. Department of Psychology, University of Haifa.

[140] Lipshitz, R., Popper, M. & Friedman, V. (2006). *Demystifying organizational learning*. Thousand Oaks, CA: Sage Publication.

[141] Pfeffer, J. & Sutton, R.I. (2006). Act on Facts, Not Faith. How management can follow medicine's lead and rely on evidence, not on half-truths. *Stanford Social Innovation Review*.

[142] Pfeffer, J. & Sutton, R.I. (2006). Hard Facts, Dangerous Half-Truths and Total Nonsense: Profiting From Evidence-Based Management. Cambridge: Harvard Business School Press.

[143] Sackett, D. L., Straus, S.E., Richardson, W.S., Rosenberg,W. & Haynes,R.B. (2000). *Evidence-based medicine: How to practice and teach EBM.* New York: Churchill Livingstone.

[144] Thomas, G. & Pring, R. (2004). *Evidence-based practice in Education.* Maidenhead: Open University Press.

[145] Rousseau, D. M. (2005). Evidence-based management in health care. In Korunka, C. and Hoffmann.P. (Eds.), *Change and quality in human service work.* Munich: Hampp Publishers.

[146] Rousseau, D. M. (2006). Is there such a thing as evidence-based management? *Acad. Manage Rev. 31*, 256-269

[147] Walshe, K. & Rundall,T.G. (2001). Evidence-based management: From theory to practice in health care. *The Milbank Quarterly. 79*, 429-457

[148] Shortell, S., Rundall,T. & Hsu,J. (2007). Improving Patient Care by Linking Evidence-Based Medicine and Evidence-Based Management. *JAMA. 298*, 673-676

[149] Berwick, D. M. (2005). Broadening the view of evidence-based medicine. *Qual. Saf. Health Care. 14*, 315-316

[150] Bradley, E., Herrin,J., Wang,Y., Barton,B., Webster,T., Mattera,J., Roumanis,S., Curtis,J., Nallamothu,B., Magid,D., McNamara,R., Parkosewich,J., Loeb,J. & Krumholz,H. (2006). Strategies for Reducing the Door-to-Balloon Time in Acute Myocardial Infarction. *N. Eng. J. Med. 355*, 2308-2320

[151] Chan, K.S., Morton, S.C. & Shekelle, P.G. (2004). Systematic Reviews for Evidence Based Management: How to Find Them and What to Do with Them. *Am. J. Manag. Care. 10*, 806-812

[152] Kovner, A.R. & Rundall, T.G. (2006). The Promise of Evidence Based Management: From Guess Work to Best Work. *Front Health Serv. Manage. 22*, 3-22

[153] Tunis, S., Stryer, D. & Clancy, C. (2003). Practical Clinical Trials: Increasing the Value of Clinical Research for Decision Making in Clinical and Health Policy. *JAMA. 290*, 1624-1632

[154] Grol, R., Berwick, D. & Wensing, M. (2008). On the trail of quality and safety in health care. *BMJ. 336*, 74-76

[155] Shortell, S. & Swartzberg, J. (2008). The Physician as Public Health Professional in the 21st Century. *JAMA. 300*, 2916-2918

[156] Nap, R.E., Andriessen, M.P.H.M., Meessen, N.E.L. & van der Werf, T.S. (2007). Pandemic Influenza and Hospital Resources. *Emerg. Infect. Dis. 13*, 1714-1719
[157] Nap R.E., Andriessen M.P.H.M., Meessen N.E.L., Miranda D.R. & van der Werf T.S. (2008). Pandemic Influenza and Excess Intensive-Care Workload. *Emerg. Infect. Dis. 14*, 1518-1525
[158] Nap, R.E., Fleer, J., Andriessen, M.P.H.M., Meessen, N.E.L. & van der Werf, T.S. (2009). Pandemic Influenza and Compliance of Health Care Workers. *Submitted.*
[159] Nap, R.E., Andriessen, M.P.H.M., Meessen, N.E.L., Albers, M.J.I.J. & van der Werf, T.S. (2009). Pandemic Influenza and Pediatric Intensive-Care. *Submitted.*
[160] Nap, R.E., Snapper, H.A., Andriessen, M.P.H.M., Meessen, N.E.L. & van der Werf, T.S. (2009). Post-Operative Care, General Medicine & Pandemic Influenza. *Submitted.*
[161] Zhang, X., Meltzer, M.I. & Wortley, P. (2005). FluSurge2.0: a manual to assist state and local public health officials and hospital administrators in estimating the impact of an influenza pandemic on hospital surge capacity (Beta test version).
[162] Centraal Bureau voor de Statistiek. (2006). *Statistisch Jaarboek 2006.* Centraal Bureau voor de Statistiek.
[163] Van Genugten, M.L.L., Heijnen, M.L.A. & Jager, J.C. (2001). Scenario ontwikkeling zorgvraag bij een influenzapandemie. *RIVM rapport 217617 004,*
[164] Miranda, D.R. (1991). Management of Resources in Intensive-Care. *Intens. Care Med. 17*, 127-128
[165] Miranda, D.R., Rivera-Fernandez, R. & Nap, R.E. (2007). Critical care medicine in the hospital: lessons from the EURICUS-studies. *Med. Intensiva. 31*, 194-203
[166] van der Werf, T.S., Zijlstra, J.G., Ligtenberg, J.J. & Tulleken, J.E. (2005). Beslissingen rond het levenseinde op de Intensive Care: overgang van curatieve naar paliatieve behandeling. *Neth. J. Med. 149*, 742-746
[167] Boussarsar, M. & Bouchoucha, S. (2006). Dying at home: cultural and religious preferences. *Intens Care Med. 32*, 1917-1918
[168] Hoare, Z. & Lim, W.S. (2006). Pneumonia: update on diagnosis and management. *BMJ. 332*, 1077-1079
[169] Seto, W.H., Tsang, D., Yung, R.W.H., Ching, T.Y., Ng, T.K., Ho, M., Ho, L.M., Peiris, J.S.M. & and Advisors of Expert SARS group of

Hospital Authority. (2003). Effectiveness of precautions against droplets and contact in prevention of nosocomial transmission of severe acute respiratory syndrome (SARS). *Lancet. 361*, 1519-1520

[170] Miranda, D.R., Nap, R., de Rijk, A., Schaufeli, W. & Iapichino, G. (2003). Nursing Activities Score. *Crit. Care Med. 31*, 374-382

[171] Swaminathan, A., Martin, R., Gamon, S., Aboltins, C., Athan, E., Braitberg, G., Catton, M.G., Cooley, L., Dwyer, D.E., Edmonds, D., Eisen, D.P., Hosking, K., Hughes, A.J., Johnson, P.D., Maclean, A.V., O'Reilly, M., Peters, S.E., Stuart, R.L., Moran, R. & Grayson, M.L. (2007). Personal Protective Equipment and Antiviral Drug Use during Hospitalization for Suspected Avian or Pandemic Influenza. *Emerg. Infect. Dis. 13*, 1541-1547

[172] Herman, B., Rosychuk, R.J., Bailey, T., Lake, R., Yonge, O. & Marrie, T.J. (2007). Medical Students and Pandemic Influenza. *Emerg. Infect. Dis. 13*, 1781-1783

[173] Bonten, M.J.M. & Prins, J.M. (2006). Antibiotics in pandemic flu. *BMJ. 332*, 248-249

[174] Christian, M. D., Hawryluck, L., Wax, R.S., Cook, T., Lazar, N.M., Herridge, M.S., Muller, M.P., Gowans, D.R., Fortier, W. & Burkle, F.M. (2006). Development of a triage protocol for critical care during an influenza pandemic. *CMAJ. 175*, 1377-1381

[175] Bulow, H.H., Sprung, C., Reinhart, K., Prayag, S., Du, B., Armaganidis, A., Abroug, F. & Levy, M. (2008). The world's major religions' points of view on end-of-life decisions in the intensive care unit. *Intens. Care Med. 34*, 423-430

[176] Sprung, C.L., Ledoux, D., Bulow, H.H., Lippert, A., Wennberg, E., Baras, M., Ricou, B., Sjokvist, P., Wallis, C., Maia, P., Thijs, L.G., Solsona, D.J. & and the ETHICUS Study Group. (2008). Relieving suffering or intentionally hastening death: Where do you draw the line? *Crit. Care Med. 36*, 8-13

INDEX

A

accountability, 45
acute, 7, 8, 40, 46, 51, 54, 58, 59, 61, 65, 70, 76, 77, 78, 81, 84, 87
acute coronary syndrome, 46
acute lung injury, 7
acute respiratory distress syndrome, 78
adaptation, 77
adjustment, 15
administrative, 57
administrators, 53, 86
adult, 61, 70
adults, 7
Africa, xi, 1, 3, 5, 8, 13, 83
age, 11, 21, 23, 28, 53, 61, 67, 76, 82
agent, 18, 25
agricultural, 29
agricultural sector, 29
agriculture, 29
aid, 70
AIDS, 7
air, 7, 41
air travel, 7
airports, 65
airways, 4
Alaska, 75
alcohol, 33
alertness, 1, 7
alternative, 28
ambulance, 37
anesthesiologists, 58
animal health, 29
animals, 8, 79
antibiotics, 6
antibody, 5, 78
antigenic drift, 4, 6
antigenic shift, 4, 6
antiviral, 7, 9, 27, 61, 65
antiviral drugs, 9, 27
antiviral therapy, 61
ARS, 40, 87
Asia, xi, 1, 3, 5, 6, 27, 28, 29, 54, 73, 74, 75, 84
Asian, xi, 1, 3, 76
Asian flu, xi, 1, 3
assessment, 38, 69
assumptions, 9, 41, 42, 69
attacks, 35, 41
Australasia, 16, 69
Australia, 6, 81
autonomy, 47
autopsy, 6
availability, 7, 16, 35
avian flu, 83
avian influenza, xi, 1, 3, 4, 6, 7, 8, 9, 17, 21, 27, 29, 67, 68, 73, 74, 75, 77, 78, 79, 80, 83, 84
awareness, 37, 41, 42, 45

B

back, 33, 35, 41, 68
bacterial, 6, 21, 65, 75
bacterial infection, 6
Barbados, 13
barriers, 17, 47
behavioral sciences, 46
beliefs, 44
benchmarking, 44
beneficial effect, 9
benefits, 29
binding, 4
bioterrorism, 82
bird flu, 79
birds, 5, 6, 7, 27, 75, 79
birth, 68
birth rate, 68
blocks, 53
blood, 6, 34
bottleneck, 54, 61
bottlenecks, 46
boys, 62
brain, 6
burn, 15

C

campaigns, 65
Canada, 40
cancer, 7, 23
care model, 45
cave, 8
CDC, 53
cell, 4, 75, 77
cell death, 75
Centers for Disease Control, 53
chickens, 1, 7
Chief of Staff, 41
children, 7, 21, 58, 61, 68, 70, 83
China, 5, 78
chronic illness, 7
citizens, 5, 39
civilian, 37, 41

classification, 80
cleaning, 33
clinics, 33
closure, 27, 65
co-existence, 27
cohort, 5
collaboration, 29, 39, 51
communication, 29, 31, 37, 39, 41, 43, 45, 51, 57, 68, 70
community, 25, 29, 37, 46, 49
co-morbidities, 63
competition, 31, 39
complexity, 35
compliance, 58
complications, 7, 9, 79
components, 9, 45, 46
confusion, 3
Congress, viii
conjunctivitis, 5, 78
constraints, 28
construction, 38
consulting, 45
contingency, 17, 80
continuity, 2, 34, 35, 49, 51, 54, 69
control, 6, 9, 27, 29, 31, 40, 76, 84
conversion, 5, 6
conversion rate, 5
COPD, 23
Coping, 76
corona, 6
corporations, 40
costs, 29
crisis management, 33, 36
critically ill, 15, 80
culture, 2, 28, 43, 44, 45, 54
cycles, 44
cytokine, 9

D

database, 69
death, 28, 75, 87
deaths, 5, 6, 12, 21, 28, 37, 75
decision makers, 41
decision making, 2, 40, 42, 43, 44

Index

decisions, 2, 33, 38, 41, 42, 43, 44, 45, 54, 59, 62, 63, 69, 70, 87
definition, 5, 40
delivery, 31, 46, 58
dentistry, 58
desert, 37
destruction, 7
detection, 6, 28, 29, 78
developing countries, 28
developing nations, 37
diabetes, 7, 23
diabetes mellitus, 23
dialysis, 33
differentiation, 36, 57, 70
disaster, 8, 17, 33, 35
disaster assistance, 38
discipline, 35, 70
discrimination, 22
diseases, 23, 36
disposables, 62
disseminate, 6
distress, 78
distribution, 11, 21, 22, 53
doctors, 6
draft, 1, 7, 40
drinking, 33
drinking water, 33
drug resistance, 25
drugs, 9, 25, 27
duties, 57, 70

E

earthquake, 36
East Asia, 29
Ebola, 8, 17
ecological, 7
ecological systems, 7
economic losses, xi, 1, 3, 51
economics, 29
ecosystem, 37
Education, 85
educators, 44
egg, 28
elderly, 7, 28, 82

eligibility criteria, 22
ELISA, 5
Emergency Department, 82
emergency management, 36
emergency response, 37
employees, 81
employment, 38
England, 75, 80
environment, 16, 22, 31, 45, 57, 70
epidemic, 17, 28, 29, 76, 77, 84
epidemics, 7, 9, 18, 83
epithelial cell, 4
epithelial cells, 4
epithelium, 77
erosion, 57
estimating, 86
ethical concerns, 44
ethics, 76, 81
Euro, 80
Europe, xi, 1, 3, 5, 6, 11, 21, 54, 81
European Commission, 78
European Union, 68
evacuation, 37
evidence-based practices, 44
evolution, 25, 79
exercise, 37
expertise, 70
exposure, 4, 70

F

failure, 1, 8, 15, 39, 81
family, 5, 17, 38, 57, 70, 81
family members, 17, 57, 70
farms, 78
fatality rates, 7
fear, 39, 42
fever, 8
fighters, 37, 41
finance, 29
financial resources, 2, 43
fire, 17, 33, 36
fire fighting, 33
fires, 35
firms, 35, 45

first responders, 37
flight, 33
flood, 36
focus group, 45
focus groups, 45
focusing, 41
food, 7, 78
food production, 7
fowl, 4
full capacity, 61
funding, 39

G

Gaza, 41
Gaza Strip, 41
gene, 4, 76, 79
general practitioner, 11, 19, 31, 39, 51, 58, 59, 63
general practitioners, 11, 19, 31, 39, 51, 58, 59, 63
generation, 21, 68, 83
genes, 4
genetic drift, 29
Geneva, 76
girls, 62
global resources, 29
government, 2, 28, 29, 36, 40, 41, 43
groups, 7, 21, 23, 27, 28, 45
Guangdong, 5, 78
Guatemala, 13
guidelines, 46, 55
guiding principles, 42
Guillain-Barré syndrome, 28

H

H1N1, 4, 83
H3N2, 4
H5N1, xi, 1, 3, 4, 6, 28, 65, 73, 74, 75, 77, 78, 80, 83
H7N4, 78
H7N7, 1, 4, 5, 7, 78
Haifa, 84

Hamas, 41
handling, 67
harbour, 8
Harvard, 85
hazards, 37
health, xi, 1, 3, 7, 8, 9, 11, 15, 16, 17, 22, 23, 27, 28, 29, 31, 33, 38, 39, 42, 43, 46, 49, 51, 53, 58, 59, 65, 67, 68, 69, 70, 76, 80, 82, 84, 85, 86
health care, xi, 1, 2, 3, 7, 9, 11, 15, 17, 23, 31, 39, 43, 46, 51, 52, 53, 58, 59, 65, 67, 68, 69, 70, 76, 85
health care professionals, 46
health care system, 2, 9, 11, 43
health care workers (HCWs), 2, 8, 9, 39, 43, 76, 81
health services, 1, 16, 22, 31, 33, 39, 43, 46, 49, 51, 52, 54, 58, 59, 67, 69, 70
healthcare, 15, 17, 27, 31, 77
heart, 23
heart disease, 23
hemagglutinin, 79
hemoglobinopathies, 7
Hezbollah, 41
high risk, 7, 9, 17
high-level, 80
high-risk, 9, 23, 65, 81
high-risk populations, 9
Hong Kong, xi, 1, 3, 5, 40, 73
hospital, 1, 2, 8, 9, 11, 12, 13, 15, 16, 17, 19, 21, 33, 39, 40, 42, 43, 49, 51, 53, 58, 59, 61, 63, 65, 67, 69, 70, 81, 86
hospital beds, 8, 13, 15, 33, 53, 61, 70
hospitalization, 8, 21, 28, 51, 82
hospitalized, 40, 67
hospitals, 1, 2, 11, 13, 15, 16, 19, 22, 31, 33, 39, 40, 43, 46, 49, 51, 54, 57, 58, 70
host, 4, 75, 77
household, 5, 40, 78
households, 40
human, xi, 1, 3, 4, 5, 7, 9, 25, 27, 29, 36, 40, 42, 46, 51, 54, 74, 77, 78, 85
human resources, 37
humanitarian, 38

Index

humans, 3, 5, 6, 27, 36, 73, 78, 80
hurricane, 36
hygiene, 7, 57

I

ICU, 9, 15, 16, 22, 51, 53, 57, 61, 63, 68, 69, 70, 80
identification, 6, 29, 37
immune response, 28, 75
immune system, 6
immunity, 3, 28, 75, 83
immunization, 28, 83
immunosuppression, 7
impact analysis, 36
implementation, 22, 36
Incidents, 35
incubation, 36
incubation period, 36
Indonesia, 5, 73
ineffectiveness, 42, 69
Infants, 79
infection, 5, 7, 9, 17, 31, 40, 65, 73, 74, 75, 80
infections, 5, 6, 78, 79, 80
infectious, xi, 1, 3, 8, 25, 75, 76
infectious disease, xi, 1, 75, 76
infectious diseases, 75, 76
inflammatory, 9
influenza, xi, 1, 3, 4, 6, 7, 8, 9, 11, 13, 16, 17, 19, 21, 23, 27, 29, 31, 35, 39, 51, 53, 58, 61, 65, 67, 68, 69, 73, 74, 75, 76, 77, 78, 79, 80, 81, 82, 83, 84, 86, 87
influenza a, 5, 6, 27, 28, 65, 74, 78, 79, 82
influenza vaccine, 27, 83
information sharing, 39, 51
information technology, 33, 45
infrastructure, 7, 36
inherited, 4
inhibition, 5, 78
inhibitor, 25
inhibitors, 21, 57
initiation, 46

injuries, 37
injury, viii, 7
Innovation, 84
inoculation, 28
insight, 36, 59, 70
institutions, 29, 40, 67, 69
insurance, 37
integration, 43, 46
integrity, 41
intensive care unit (ICU), 40, 53, 80, 81, 87
intentions, 41
internet, 28, 69
interview, 53, 61
intoxication, 8
isolation, 6, 25, 65
Israel, 41, 84
Italy, 78

J

JAMA, 82, 85
Japan, 82
justice, 22, 37

K

kidnapping, 41
knowledge transfer, 45

L

land, 37, 41
land-use, 37
language, 35, 44
law, 36, 39, 44
law enforcement, 44
leadership, 29, 45
learning, 35, 44, 45, 84
Lebanon, 41, 84
legislation, 37
levees, 37
likelihood, 28
limitations, 25, 67

linear, 53
linkage, 45
liver, 1, 6, 8
liver failure, 1, 8
location, 42
long-distance, 78
losses, 1, 3, 42, 51
lung, 7

M

magnetic, viii
maintenance, 37
mammals, 6
management, 1, 2, 8, 33, 35, 39, 42, 43, 44, 45, 46, 47, 51, 52, 55, 61, 65, 69, 70, 74, 84, 85, 86
management practices, 35, 46
manpower, 31, 81
market, 45
Maryland, 17
matrix, 79
measurement, 70
measures, 6, 27, 29, 31, 36, 40, 58, 65, 84
mechanical ventilation, 9, 16
medical care, 8, 43, 46, 54, 61
medical school, 51
medical student, 58
medication, 65
medications, 7, 65
memory, 38
men, 40
messages, 51
migration, 5
military, 38
models, 2, 9, 11, 27, 28, 43, 51, 59, 65, 67, 68, 69
molecules, 4
morale, 40, 57, 68
morbidity, 9, 15, 17, 23, 25, 84
morning, 33
mortality, 3, 5, 6, 9, 11, 15, 17, 21, 22, 23, 54, 65, 68, 76, 80
mortality rate, 3, 15

movement, 58
mutation, 6, 73
mutations, 4
myocardial infarction, 46

N

NEMS, 68, 81
Netherlands, 1, 2, 5, 7, 8, 11, 12, 15, 17, 19, 21, 23, 49, 51, 53, 58, 59, 61, 65, 67, 71, 78, 80, 82
neuraminidase, 21, 25, 57, 76
neurosurgery, 15
New York, vii, viii, 17, 85
New Zealand, 81
next generation, 83
NHS, 22
non-clinical, 17
normal, 33, 54, 57
norms, 40
North America, 6
nucleoprotein, 79
nurse, 15
nurses, 2, 43, 45, 53, 57, 62, 77
nursing, 7, 11, 15, 31, 39, 44, 49, 51, 55, 68, 70, 81
nursing home, 7, 11, 31, 39, 49, 51

O

oat, 3
obligation, 18
obligations, 17, 81
observations, 21
occupational, 5
on-line, 69
organ, 6, 15, 81
organizational culture, 44, 45
orientation, 41
Oseltamivir, 83
outpatient, 34
outpatients, 33
overload, 19
oversight, 36

P

pandemic, xi, 1, 3, 6, 7, 9, 11, 12, 16, 17, 19, 21, 22, 23, 25, 27, 29, 31, 35, 39, 51, 53, 57, 58, 61, 63, 65, 67, 68, 69, 70, 73, 74, 75, 76, 79, 80, 81, 82, 83, 84, 86, 87
Pandemic Influenza Preparedness, 79
pathogenic, 4, 5, 73, 78, 83
pathogens, 65
patient care, 17, 33, 69
patient management, 2, 52, 55, 61
patients, 1, 5, 7, 8, 11, 12, 13, 15, 16, 17, 19, 21, 22, 33, 36, 39, 40, 43, 46, 54, 57, 58, 59, 61, 65, 67, 68, 69, 70, 79, 80, 81
pediatric, 21, 61, 62
peer, 44
perceptions, 82
personal values, 40
pharmaceutical, 25
pharmacological, 74
physicians, 15, 18, 45, 46, 47, 49, 53, 57, 77, 81
Physicians, 70, 82
physiological, 22
planning, xi, 1, 9, 17, 21, 29, 31, 35, 42, 43, 51, 57, 67, 70, 79, 81
play, 11, 17, 19, 31, 59
pneumonia, 6, 16, 21, 54, 65, 75, 79
police, 17, 37
policymakers, 29
polymerase, 4, 77
population, 4, 6, 7, 8, 9, 11, 19, 21, 23, 27, 28, 33, 37, 40, 53, 57, 59, 68, 70
poultry, 1, 5, 7, 28, 67, 78
power, 33, 38, 41
prediction, 37
preference, 47
preparedness, xi, 1, 7, 17, 21, 29, 31, 37, 43, 51, 67, 69, 80, 82, 84
pressure, 44, 55
prevention, 35, 87
priming, 84
prisoners, 41
probability, 29, 37
production, 7, 25, 27, 33
professionalism, 57, 77
program, 53, 83
pro-inflammatory, 9
property rights, 28
prophylactic, 25, 57
protection, 4, 9, 29, 36, 57, 65
protein, 3
protocol, 87
protocols, 55, 57, 65
prototype, 44, 83
public, 3, 9, 11, 15, 16, 17, 22, 27, 28, 31, 33, 37, 39, 41, 42, 49, 51, 52, 54, 58, 65, 67, 69, 70, 82, 86
public awareness, 37
public health, 3, 9, 15, 16, 22, 27, 28, 31, 33, 39, 42, 49, 51, 52, 54, 58, 67, 69, 70, 82, 86
public opinion, 41
public service, 3, 17

Q

quality improvement, 46
quarantine, 1, 8, 25, 27, 36, 65
query, 83
questioning, 45
questionnaire, 58

R

range, 15, 16, 42
reactivity, 83
reading, 44
recognition, 43, 69
recovery, 35
recruiting, 45
regional, 1, 2, 7, 8, 31, 35, 39, 43, 51, 69
regular, 53, 61
rehearsing, 38
relationships, 45
relatives, 57, 63, 68
relevance, 41

religions, 87
renal, 7
renal dysfunction, 7
repair, 38
reparation, 31
resilience, 68
resistance, 25, 82
resources, 2, 13, 15, 16, 22, 23, 28, 29, 35, 43, 45, 47, 51, 61, 67, 70, 80, 81
respiratory, 4, 15, 65, 76, 77, 78, 81, 84, 87
respiratory distress syndrome, 78
respiratory failure, 15
returns, 77, 79
risk, 1, 7, 9, 17, 21, 23, 28, 35, 46, 65, 67, 70, 81
risk assessment, 37
risk management, 35
risks, 17, 28, 37, 41, 44
rural, 27, 29
rural areas, 27
rural development, 29

S

safety, 79, 85
SARS, xi, 1, 3, 6, 17, 36, 40, 57, 65, 76, 77, 84, 86
scalable, 35
scarce resources, 13, 22, 70
Scenario Analysis, 80
school, 25, 27, 51, 65
search, 38, 83
search engine, 83
Second World, 75
security, 33
Security Council, 42
sepsis, 9, 16, 54
services, viii, xi, 1, 2, 3, 7, 11, 15, 16, 17, 22, 23, 31, 33, 37, 39, 43, 46, 49, 51, 52, 53, 58, 59, 65, 67, 68, 69, 70, 80
settlements, 41
severe acute respiratory syndrome, 76, 81, 84, 87

severity, 15
sewage, 38
sharing, 31, 39, 51
shock, 15
shortage, 58, 61
shortages, 41
side effects, 44
simulation, 16
Singapore, 57, 84
sites, 36
smallpox, 17
social environment, 57
social network, 27
social standing, 41
social systems, xi, 1, 3, 51
socioeconomic, 84
South Africa, 83
South America, 13
Southeast Asia, 27, 74
Southern Hemisphere, 79
Spanish flu, xi, 1, 3, 28
species, 4, 8
sporadic, 74
staffing, 15
standard operating procedures, 40
statistics, 35
stock, 5, 65
stockpile, 25, 27, 29
stockpiling, 25, 37
strain, 3, 5, 16, 21, 22, 23, 28, 29, 31, 58, 63, 70
strains, 6, 29
strategies, 27, 37, 45, 46, 84
strikes, 37
students, 58
sub-Saharan Africa, 8
suffering, xi, 1, 3, 40, 51, 87
Sumatra, 5
summaries, 44
supply, 28, 33, 42
surgeons, 58
surgery, 15, 54
surgical, 8, 58, 70
surveillance, 7, 27, 29, 40
survival, 35, 52

Index

susceptibility, 75
Switzerland, 76
symptoms, 1, 6, 8, 46
syndrome, 28, 76, 77, 78, 81, 84, 87

T

tanks, 33
team members, 36, 55
Tel Aviv, 42
telephone, 53, 61
terrorism, 36
therapy, 51, 61
thinking, 2
thoracic, 15, 58
thoracic surgeon, 58
threat, 7, 29, 36, 39, 41, 74, 80
threats, 36, 47
throat, 6
time periods, 42
time pressure, 47, 55
toxic, 1, 8
trade, 7
training, 15, 37, 39, 40, 51, 53, 57, 58, 70
trans, 5
transfer, 45
transformation, 53
transmission, 3, 5, 29, 40, 54, 73, 76, 77, 80, 87
transparency, 41
transparent, 36
transplant, 7
trauma, 1, 8, 11, 33, 39
travel, 7, 25, 40
triage, 19, 22, 39, 46, 51, 59, 62, 63, 70, 87
trial, 79, 83
tropism, 4
trucks, 33
Tuberculosis, 2

U

Uganda, 1, 8
uncertain outcomes, 40
uncertainty, 1, 3, 8, 77
undergraduate, 58
United Kingdom, 15, 16, 69
United Nations, 28
United States, 7, 13, 15, 18, 75, 82
universities, 45

V

vaccination, 9, 25, 27, 28, 65, 83
vaccine, 9, 25, 27, 28, 40, 65, 82, 83, 84
validation, 35
values, 40, 44
variables, 15, 68
ventilation, 9, 16
victims, 3, 6
village, 5
virological, 5
virulence, 4
virus, xi, 1, 3, 4, 6, 7, 9, 25, 27, 29, 65, 73, 74, 75, 76, 77, 78, 79, 83, 84
virus infection, 73, 79
viruses, 4, 6, 7, 73, 77, 78, 82, 83
visible, 45
vulnerability, 37

W

Wales, 75
war, 8, 39, 40, 42
waste disposal, 33
water, 4, 33, 38
waterfowl, 4, 78
welfare, 33
WHO, 7, 21, 25, 28, 54, 67, 70, 73, 74, 75
wildlife, 4, 78
workers, 2, 8, 9, 17, 31, 37, 39, 43, 76, 81, 82
workflow, 46

workforce, 57
workload, 57, 68, 70, 81
workplace, 25
World Health Organisation, 73

World Health Organization (WHO), 1, 7, 74, 75, 77, 82